MW00413713

Lean-Six Sigma for Healthcare

Also available from ASQ Quality Press:

Stop Rising Healthcare Costs Using Toyota Lean Production Methods: 38 Steps for Improvement
Robert Chalice

The Manager's Guide to Six Sigma in Healthcare: Practical Tips and Tools for Improvement
Robert Barry and Amy C. Smith

Nan: A Six Sigma Mystery
Robert Barry

Measuring Quality Improvement in Healthcare: A Guide to Statistical Process Control Applications
Raymond G. Carey, Ph.D. and Robert C. Lloyd, Ph.D.

The Six Sigma Book for Healthcare: Improving Outcomes by Reducing Errors
Robert Barry, Ph.D.; Amy Murcko, APRN; and Clifford Brubaker, Ph.D.

Improving Healthcare with Control Charts: Basic and Advanced SPC Methods and Case Studies
Raymond G.Carey

The Six Sigma Journey from Art to Science
Larry Walters

Six Sigma for the Office: A Pocket Guide
Roderick Munro

Defining and Analyzing a Business Process: A Six Sigma Pocket Guide
Jeffrey N. Lowenthall

Customer Centered Six Sigma: Linking Customers, Process Improvement, and Financial Results
Earl Naumann and Steven H. Hoisington

Office Kaizen: Transforming Office Operations Into a Strategic Competitive Advantage
William Lareau

To request a complimentary catalog of ASQ Quality Press publications, call 800-248-1946, or visit our website at http://qualitypress.asq.org .

Lean-Six Sigma for Healthcare

A Senior Leader Guide to Improving
Cost and Throughput

Chip Caldwell, FACHE
Jim Brexler, FACHE
Tom Gillem

ASQ Quality Press
Milwaukee, Wisconsin

American Society for Quality, Quality Press, Milwaukee 53203

© 2005 by American Society for Quality

All rights reserved. Published 2005

Printed in the United States of America

12 11 10 09 08 07 06   5 4 3 2

Library of Congress Cataloging-in-Publication Data

Caldwell, Chip.
  Lean-Six Sigma for healthcare : a senior leader guide to improving cost and
    throughput / Chip Caldwell, Jim Brexler, Tom Gillem.
      p. cm.
  Includes bibliographical references and index.
  ISBN 0-87389-647-5 (hardback : alk. paper)
  1. Health services administration—Quality control.   2. Medical care—
  Cost-effectiveness.   3. Six sigma (Quality control standard)
  4. Organizational effectiveness.   5. Performance standards.   6. Strategic
  planning.   7. Chief executive officers.   8. Hospital administrators.
  I. Brexler, Jim.   II. Gillem, Tom.   III. Title.

  RA399.A1C345 2005
  362.1'068—dc22   2005005208

ISBN 0-87389-647-5

Publisher: William A. Tony
Acquisitions Editor: Annemieke Hytinen
Project Editor: Paul O'Mara
Production Administrator: Randall Benson

Extend screen captures courtesy of Imagine That, Inc. of San Jose, CA. Extend is a
trademark of Imagine That, Inc.

ASQ Mission: The American Society for Quality advances individual,
organizational, and community excellence worldwide through learning, quality
improvement, and knowledge exchange.

Attention Bookstores, Wholesalers, Schools, and Corporations: ASQ Quality Press
books, videotapes, audiotapes, and software are available at quantity discounts
with bulk purchases for business, educational, or instructional use. For
information, please contact ASQ Quality Press at 800-248-1946, or write to ASQ
Quality Press, P.O. Box 3005, Milwaukee, WI 53201-3005.

To place orders or to request a free copy of the ASQ Quality Press Publications
Catalog, including ASQ membership information, call 800-248-1946. Visit our
Web site at www.asq.org or http://qualitypress.asq.org.

∞ Printed on acid-free paper

Quality Press
600 N. Plankinton Avenue
Milwaukee, Wisconsin 53203
Call toll free 800-248-1946
Fax 414-272-1734
www.asq.org
http://qualitypress.asq.org
http://standardsgroup.asq.org
E-mail: authors@asq.org

AMERICAN SOCIETY
FOR QUALITY™

To all who seek to serve God and others, in their professional and personal missions.

—Chip Caldwell

To my wife, Sharon, who has been a constant source of inspiration and encouragement to me throughout our marriage and my career.

—Jim Brexler

To my wife, Anne, and our daughter, Beth, whose love and support make my world a wonderful place.

—Tom Gillem

Contents

CD Contents

The CD is organized for maximum utility by the following attributes:

- By Role
- By Focus Area or Question
- By Book Chapter

The tools and learning labs listed below can also be downloaded, along with updated cases and articles, from www.chipcaldwellassoc.com/resources.html

Readers who access the tools, slides, and learning lab suggestions can search by any or all of the organizational categories for ease of use and purpose.

By Role	By Focus Area or Question	By Book Chapter
CEO/COO/Senior Leaders	**Cost Improvement**	**Chapter 1**
What is the CEO/ COO role in Lean-Six Sigma strategy deployment? • Scan the Preface, particularly CEO Lowell Kruse comments, and Chapters 2 & 3. • Conduct CEO Role Self-Assessment. • Where can we acquire aggressive benchmarks?	We need $1 million removed quickly. What is the most effective method? 100-Day Waste Workout • Waste Walk sample agenda and facilitator instructions • Slides for session. • Waste Walk idea generator • Where can we acquire aggressive benchmarks?	• DMAIC Charter Example • Balanced Scorecard for Lean-Six Sigma • Belief System Transformation Session Sample Agenda (with facilitator instructions, room layout, and handouts.) (Also referred to by its method – Appreciative Inquiry, discussed in Chapter 6.)

Continued

By Role	By Focus Area or Question	By Book Chapter

• We need to reduce $1 million quickly. What is the most effective method? 100-Day Waste Workout
 	
–Reread Chapter 2 and the 100-Day Workout method in Chapter 3.
 	
–Waste Walk instructions
 	
–Slides for session
 	
–Waste Walk idea generator fo. manager breakout session
 	
–If cost is an issue and comparative benchmarks will accelerate your efforts, acquire aggressive benchmarks.
 	
• How do we set up a multi-year results and project tracking system?
 	
  • Rreread the Magic Moment section of Chapter 4.
 	
  • EXCELerator™ online tracking system
 	
  • Magic Moment spreadsheet for the COO & CFO to layout multi-year goals, projects, and tracking.
 	
  • If cost goal-setting is an issue, acquire comparative data.
 	
• How do we get all departments involved in cost and throughput improvement?
 	
  • Conduct Senior Leader Learning Lab on Engaging Physicians.
	• How is a 100-Day Waste Workout conducted?
	
	–100-Day Waste Workout agenda
	
	–Waste Walk idea generator
	
	–Session Slides
	
	Strategic Measurement
	
	• How do we set up a multi-year results project tracking system?
	
	–EXCELerator™ online tracking system
	
	–Magic Moment spreadsheet
	
	• How do we upgrade our current strategic measurement template or balanced scorecard?
	
	Software and Online Tools
	
	• What software is best for Lean-Six Sigma DMAIC projects?
	
	–Download 3-day free trial of MINITAB™ statistical package.
	
	–Learn about Quality Companion for project guidance.
	
	• What is best for 100-Day Workout results tracking?
	
	–EXCELerator™
	
	Culture/Belief System
	
	• We are not sure our culture is ready for aggressive cost & throughput improvement. How can we assess our readiness?
	
	• We know we have less "will" to implement than we need. What can we do to strengthen our resolve?
		• PDCA Method Assessment Template
		
		• 100-Day Workout Agenda template
		
		(See also Waste Walk document in Chapter 2.)
		
		• Learning Lab: 1-hour Senior Leader Session to dialogue current approaches of assuring projects are strategic versus tactical.
		
		Chapter 2
		
		• In-Quality / Out-of Quality Staffing Workshop Facilitation slides
		
		• DMAIC Project Charter template
		
		• Waste Walk idea generator
		
		• Lean-Six Sigma Solution Set
		
		• Glossary
		
		• Learning Lab: Manager "In Quality" / "Out of Quality" Staffing Dialogue
		
		• Learning Lab: Senior Leader Waste Walk to learn to coach managers in removing process waste.
		
		• Learning Lab: Manager Waste Walk to generate ideas for Cost of Quality recovery.
		
		• (Note: If converting ideas from the Waste Walk are important, conduct a 100-Day Waste Workout de-scribed in Chapter 2.)
		
		–Waste Walk sample agenda and facilitator instructions

Continued

By Role	By Focus Area or Question	By Book Chapter
• Magic Moment multi-year planning spreadsheet • Process Strategic Goal-Setting Workshop to set process-specific goals that drive Cost of Quality recovery. • Waste Walk to generate creative short-term goals for managers. • How do we get physicians involved? • Conduct Senior Leader Learning Lab on Engaging Physicians. • Culture and belief system transformation is vital to the success of any initiative like Lean-Six Sigma. How can I assure that we are focusing on culture requirements as well as, the technical side? • Conduct the Belief System Transformation Session Sample Agenda, facilitator guide, room layout, and handouts.) • How do we know that we are ready to deploy Lean-Six Sigma methods and strategy? • Conduct the Lean-Six Sigma Readiness Assessment. • Then, conduct the Senior Leader Learning Lab to assess current approaches.		–Slides for session. –Waste Walk idea generator • (Note: If comparative benchmarks are needed to set goals, acquire benchmarks.) **Chapter 3** • Magic Moment Planner spreadsheet for laying out multi-year projects • Cost Goal to Process Goal Translation Workshop • CEO Role in Lean-Six Sigma Deployments – a self-assessment • Learning Lab: Senior Leader Session to assess current methods' effectiveness **Chapter 4** • Learning Lab: Senior Leader translate cost goals into process goals for strategic project deployment **Chapter 5** • Learning Lab: Senior Leaders learning the role of simulation in Lean-Six Sigma **Chapter 6** • Appreciative Inquiry Agenda and Facilitator Instructions **Chapter 7** • Learning Lab: Engaging Physicians

Continued

Continued

By Role	By Focus Area or Question	By Book Chapter
• Measurement is also vitally important. How should we think about strategic metrics and balanced scorecarding when deploying Lean-Six Sigma?		
• What education and learning sessions can we extract from the book? (Learning Labs for Senior Leaders and Managers)		

Black Belts/ Quality Professionals/ Education
 	
• I/ we have been asked to construct senior leader training in Lean-Six Sigma. What training should senior leaders receive?
 	
  • Are our current methods strategic or tactical?
  • How can we learn to coach managers in Waste? (Senior Leader Waste Walk)
  • How can we lead managers in a Waste Walk?
 	
    –Waste Walk instructions
    –Slides
    –Waste Walk idea generator
 	
• Where do we learn "Lean-Six Sigma" terminology?
• What criteria should be included in a good project charter?
• Where do I learn more? (Bibliography)
• How is a 100-Day Waste Workout conducted?
 	
  • 100-Day Waste Workout agenda
  • Waste Walk idea generator
  • Session Slides
	Current Quality System Effectiveness
	
	• How do we assess the effectiveness of our current methods?	

Figures and Tables

FIGURES

Source: Chip Caldwell & Associates, LLC. Reprinted with permission.

TABLES

Preface

This book was written specifically for CEOs, the "O-Suite," and senior leaders who desire to harness the power of Lean-Six Sigma as their major strategic weapon for progress, as well as those charged to coach them. It is intended for organizations that operate active Lean-Six Sigma initiatives but have yet to successfully attack high-leverage processes, such as "In Quality Staffing" and recovering significant Cost of Quality from throughput improvements. It is also intended for senior leaders who have yet to tackle Lean-Six Sigma as their major organizationwide strategic weapon.

However, this book is a "must read" for managers at all levels, quality professionals, and Lean-Six Sigma Black Belts who want to help ensure that their organizations' improvement efforts attack strategically versus the all-too-common tactical, project-by-project approach that suboptimizes the power of Lean-Six Sigma. Further, the book, accompanying CD, and supporting website are full of checklists, tools, templates, suggestions for additional reading, and recommended 1-hour and 2-hour learning sessions for senior leaders and managers.

Second, what is the best use of this book? The authors devoted significant effort to enable senior leaders to advance their organizations to the next level through disciplined application, as follows:

1. Read the book to digest new concepts and to incorporate those new or enhanced concepts into their existing Lean-Six Sigma thinking.

2. Create a yearlong senior leader and manager Learning Lab by going back to the Recommended Learning Session segments contained in the book and systemically deploying advanced learning opportunities for the senior leadership and for directors and managers.

3. Conduct a detailed quality system assessment (template provided in Chapter 3 and on the CD), seeking to discover the strengths and shortfalls of current approaches and methods and charting the course to the next level.

4. Incorporate as many of the tools, templates, and checklists as they can into the existing quality system, approaches, and methods.

5. Commit to share lessons learned from activities stimulated through this book and other media to capture further advancements in the field.

The first question a senior leader may likely ask upon picking up this book might be, "Why should I read this book?" It's a worthy question, particularly if posed by a busy senior leader whose main role may not be the introduction and innovation of more advanced methods contained in the organization's quality system.

The elements of lean thinking and Six Sigma can be driven only by the senior leaders of the organization. As Don Berwick, MD, president of the Institute for Healthcare Improvement in Boston and an undisputed world leader in quality system evolution, has stated, "Senior leaders today must learn to coach in the actual methods of (care)" (Berwick 1996). He further observed that past attempts to delegate major care system redesign to physicians and middle managers, those who do not see the organization from a senior leader mind-set, have largely failed because middle managers are not equipped to implement the system of care that is needed for major change. This task of system redesign is, in his words, "a nondelegable role of senior leaders."

To aid in this quest, this book will attempt to provide senior leaders with the following insights:

- How can Lean-Six Sigma aggressively improve throughput and quality while extracting significant costs within the organization?

- What is Lean, what is Six Sigma, and what are their relationships to productivity, process waste, and cost structures?

- How can a sophisticated quality system such as Lean-Six Sigma be used to achieve long-term strategic results versus simply using a project-by-project tactical approach?

- How might we adapt our existing infrastructure to take maximum strategic advantage of the power of Lean-Six Sigma?

- What is the role of senior leaders in laying out a long-term Lean-Six Sigma strategy, and how can we track results over time to ensure that goals are achieved?

- Does our organization have the capacity for change and competency to achieve our strategic goals?

It is *not* an aim of this book to rehash material contained in the excellent manuals that exist or to provide quality professionals with a how-to Lean-Six Sigma Black Belt project manual. Our purpose is decidedly strategic and from a senior leader point of view.

However, this book is a must-read for all quality professionals, financial analysts, Black Belts, managers, and physician leaders to ensure that their roles synergize with the strategic mind-set of senior leaders. Moreover, numerous references, checklists, tools, and recommended learning sessions will be provided at the end of each chapter for senior leaders, quality professionals, and others who want to learn Black Belt skills.

Successful Lean-Six Sigma deployment begins and ends with a focus on achieving strategic results. That statement alone should be enough to pique the interest of senior leaders who, in most healthcare organizations, are charged with accomplishing that very challenge—achieving strategic results.

One major flaw that occurs when Lean-Six Sigma is deployed in many healthcare organizations is that although some organizations allocate resources to launch Lean-Six Sigma programs, few organizations meet the criteria for the strategic deployment of Lean-Six Sigma. More troubling is the fact that many of these organizations do not even recognize that they approach Lean-Six Sigma tactically. Rather, these deployments are unknowingly tactical; that is, when asked to describe their programs, senior leaders begin their answers with methodology, the resources required, and the results of projects completed.

In the pages that follow, we encourage senior leaders to embark on a journey of sorts—one that will, if we achieve our objectives, take leaders down a different path in the exploration and implementation of methods that drive quantum improvement. The chapters that follow will address:

- Lean and Six Sigma concepts that equip senior leaders to *coach* managers and others in the actual methods of improvement and to enlighten even highly skilled quality professionals in transforming the existing quality system, even if Lean-Six Sigma projects have been under way for some time, into a robust strategic approach.

- The relationship between process performance and avoidable cost such as Cost of Quality and Cost of Poor Quality and techniques to ensure the recovery of these costs.

- Strategy deployment concepts, tools, methods, and approaches that ensure that Lean-Six Sigma projects are maximally aligned over time.

- The roles of senior leaders and other key players in a vibrant Lean-Six Sigma strategy.

- Effective Lean-Six Sigma strategy deployment infrastructure issues.

- Specific questions and issues that senior leaders should address with Lean-Six Sigma project leaders and quality professionals—requirements such as the criteria to be contained in every project charter, critical-process root-cause correlation techniques, and the effective use of small-scale experiments to ensure that process changes truly drive overall results.

- The various roles, responsibilities, and accountabilities that must be present to optimize the strategic power of Lean-Six Sigma.

Each chapter concludes with checklists and tools available on the accompanying CD, lists of Internet-based resources, references for further reading, and suggested learning sessions for senior leader and manager learning sessions to hardwire application throughout the organization.

Finally, throughout the book, two graphic images appear at critical points to flag the reader's attention.

The first of these, a lightbulb, is placed to slow the reader's pace and highlight a concept we believe is vital to senior leaders interested in optimizing the material.

The second, a hammer, signifies a reader-accessible tool that can be found in the appendices, on the CD, or online. At the end of each chapter, a section called "Checklists and Tools Accessible Electronically" provides sources and/or locations for tools the readers can use within their organizations or to build education sessions for others. Many of the tools are contained in the appendices, while others are precrafted PowerPoint presentations, Excel spreadsheets, PDF files, or Word templates available on the CD or for downloading at www.chipcaldwellassoc.com; click on Resources.

The following chapter outline prepares the reader for topics that will follow. While these topics have been arranged to convey a logical, practical, and applicable order, readers are encouraged to move throughout the book in nonsequential fashion to meet their specific or immediate needs, or to ask a staff person or colleague to review and report to the senior leader team on a particular concept. In fact, the "Learning Session for a Senior Leader Meeting" section at the end of many chapters is intended to enable senior leader team learning. To ensure that topics in later chapters are fully optimized, however, the reader or facilitator is encouraged to digest each chapter's major concepts, highlighted with the lightbulb.

 Finally, before beginning Chapter 1, readers might benefit from a cursory review of the Glossary. While attempting to fully comprehend all terms is not a desirable or perhaps even a possible goal, understanding terms is a bit of a chicken-and-egg issue. Which should come first? It has been our experience that a brief overview of terms that will be raised during the course of Lean-Six Sigma apprenticing increases retention, comprehension, applicability, and the natural overload that occurs when attempting to master a new language such as Lean-Six Sigma.

REFERENCES

Berwick, Donald. 1996. *Run to Space.* Video. Boston: Institute for Healthcare Improvement.

Acknowledgments

We extend our deepest appreciation and gratitude to many, many individuals and learning organizations that have made possible the compilation of the ideas, concepts, case studies, tools, and methods presented in this book. Among those most deserving of acknowledgement are:

- Dave Ferrin, for his significant contribution as a chapter author on the effective use of simulation in a Lean-Six Sigma environment. Marty Miller, Dave's colleague, for his instrumental contribution to case study development, education, and results achieved.

- Bruce Tilley, managing principal, Lean-Six Sigma Productivity Group, Chip Caldwell Associates, for his insightful innovation of Lean-Six Sigma application to processes that drive productivity and cost recovery, particularly those that aid managers in defining and managing to a high level of performance, "In Quality Staffing" and "Out of Quality Staffing," and in the application of these breakthrough constructs to demand scheduling, demand leveling, and staff scheduling processes. Further, Bruce has taken the Waste Walk method initially piloted by Sherry Bright, and the accompanying 100-Day Workout method, to highly productive levels. In addition to adding significant productivity-enhancing constructs to the Waste Walk, Bruce created two additional methods—Rapid Cycle Productivity Variance Response and Quality Staffing—to make up the 100-Day Workout Productivity Series.

- Lynne Sisak, BSN, MBA, Master Black Belt, for her brilliant work in throughput and flow optimization techniques and the optimization of "In Quality" and "Out of Quality" staffing discovery. Furthermore, Lynne has been instrumental in advancing the metrics required for effective project chartering and senior leader championing for quantifying Cost of Quality recovery as a direct relationship and correlation to dependent process throughput improvement.

- Greg Butler, EVP, Chip Caldwell Associates, for his translation of very complex engineering, statistical, and project management applications into understandable, deployable, and sustainable methods, tools, and training that can be maximized by committed senior leadership teams.

- Arvind Salvekar, Ph.D., Master Black Belt, for his insights into flow discovery, including the development and refinement of the 14-day longitudinal study methodology. This method has been instrumental in aiding project leaders and senior leader champions in understanding which subprocesses will drive toward process and system goals.

- Sherry Bright, for her piloting and innovating the first version of the Waste Walk technique, which has enabled countless organizations, senior leaders, managers, and Black Belts to discover and systematically recover the Cost of Quality from waste.

- To Chuck MacFarlane, vice president, American College of Healthcare Executives, for his support over the past eight years in enabling us to take to senior leaders the "Good to Great in Healthcare" lessons and our popular course, "Aggressively Improve Cost and Throughput Using Lean-Six Sigma." Access to leading healthcare leaders has enabled us to extract many lessons and teaching suggestions from dialogue around these sometimes complex topics.

- To clients and friends Michael McEachern, executive vice president, Sisters of Charity Providence Hospitals; Phil Beauchamp, CEO, Lisa Johnson, senior vice president, patient care, Dr. Brian Cook, and Donna Moran, all of Morton Plant Health System; Lee Huntley, CEO, Ricardo Forbes, COO, and Jill Symanski, Black Belt, all of Miami Baptist Health System; Barry Ronan, CEO, and Kim Repac, CFO, all of Western Maryland Health System; John Grah, Scripps Health System; Phillip Clendenin, CEO, and Kevin Cook, COO and Black Belt, both of River Region Health System; Lowell Kruse, CEO, senior leaders Rudy Wacker, Curt Kretzinger, Lisa Michaelis, Dottie Bray, Kaye Stegar, and Black Belt Mike Dittamore, all currently or formally of Heartland Health; Gary Muller, CEO, and Erie Hebert, executive vice president, both of West Jefferson Health System; and Darlene Delancey, Black Belt Ro Hurley, and Mary-Ellen Piche, all of the Veterans Administration Health System of Upstate New York.

- Carol Gilhooley, Joint Commission on Accreditation of Healthcare Organizations, director of survey methods development, for aid in cross-walking flow accreditation standards to the strategic application of Lean-Six Sigma.

- Harry Hertz head of the Baldrige National Quality Award team at the National Institute of Standards and Technology for his aid in relating Lean-Six Sigma as a quality system to the Baldrige Framework.

- Tom Day, president, Healthcare Management Council, one of the nation's leading comparative data companies, and his staff for their incisive analysis of quantum improvers and nonstarters on our joint Good to Great in Healthcare research over the past three years.

- I, Jim Brexler, would like to thank the following people, who have played a vital role in my professional development leading to the publishing of this book: Jim Albright, for giving me my first position in healthcare management and being my mentor; Gene Beyt and Sherry Bright, for introducing me to the philosophy and concepts of total quality management; Bill Jenkins and the late Merv Trail, for supporting my interest in teaching; Chip Caldwell, for being my coach, friend, collaborator, and colleague; and finally the executives, managers, supervisors, quality directors, physicians, and staff who have demonstrated to me the power of the tools and principles reflected in this book by putting them into practice.

- Annemieke Hytinen and Paul O'Mara of ASQ.

- And, finally, Tom Nolan, whose original thinking on change concepts and rapid cycle experiments continues to enlighten us all.

1

The Role of Senior Leaders: Raising the Performance Bar

Lucy: "Do you think anybody ever really changes?"

Linus: "I've changed a lot in the last year."

Lucy: "I meant for the better."

Charles Schultz

owell Kruse, longtime CEO of nationally recognized Heartland Health in St. Joseph, Missouri, gets it—and the point is made by such results as winning a Missouri Quality Award, being among the top 150 hospitals in clinical outcomes by Healthgrades, sustaining top-quartile productivity for several years running, and receiving too many quality team awards to list. "To be effective, any quality system, whether it's Six Sigma or the next generation of advanced methods, must be owned and managed by the executive team as a strategic tool, not deployed so low into the organization that activities become tactical," remarked Lowell in explaining the role of quality systems in quantum improver organizations (Caldwell 2004a). He further said that executive leaders must not just manage the methods contained in the Six Sigma suite, but, more importantly, must also ensure excellence in the truly critical aspects of Lean-Six Sigma. An orderly progression to ensure the strategic deployment of a Lean-Six Sigma initiative suggests the following three elements:

- Strategically aligning the executive team into a strategic steering body, not to select projects, as has been recommended by so many Six Sigma enthusiasts (Pande 2000), but rather to:

  – Determine the one-year and three-year results that must be realized in order to meet the organization's strategies.

  – Translate outcome and cost goals into process goals as a basis for Lean-Six Sigma deployment.

1

- Maintain an organizationwide, integrated system map highlighting the interrelationships between goals and leaders of core processes such as patient care throughput, emergency department, registration, and laboratory.

- Assign each key strategy to a single accountable executive.

- Allocate Six Sigma resources, called Black Belts, not globally to the entire executive team or, worse, lower into the organization, but rather to each accountable executive, who is empowered to engage her managers and other process owners in high-leverage Six Sigma projects aimed at achievement of her strategies.

- Measure through advanced scorecarding techniques progress along the way, particularly detecting results slippage so that immediate remedial action can be crafted by the executive in charge.

- Establish a monthly milestone tracking process that serves as an early warning system so that the effectiveness of remedial action can be tested.

 Heartland Health refers to the above infrastructure as the "Magic Moment," a term coined by chief operating officer Curt Kretzinger to establish with great clarity the long-term strategic results required and the deployed infrastructure to support its achievement.

By applying this disciplined process and structure, as will be discussed in Chapter 8, "The Role of Senior Leaders: Achieving Sustainable Results," national award-winning Morton Plant Hospital in Clearwater, FL, drove emergency department (ED) satisfaction from the 61st percentile to beyond the 90th percentile, a 50% improvement, while dropping ED length of stay by 25% and recovering over $4 million in Cost of Quality (COQ).

- Conducting continuous applied learning for the executive team in order to convert Six Sigma theory into practical, deployable action and measurable, sustainable bottom-line results. As former General Electric (GE) CEO Jack Welch told a group of hospital CEOs (Caldwell 2004b), the role of senior leaders is to sponsor learning activities and "rapidly convert that learning into action." At Heartland, one member of the executive team reports on a leading management or Six Sigma topic each month, addressing several questions: "What are the key take-home messages from this research?" "How are these lessons applicable to Heartland Health?" and "What action, if any, should we take now to hardwire these lessons throughout Heartland Health?"

- Engaging in purposeful executive-driven activities to reshape the organization's culture from one that accepts "error and waste as an unavoidable by-product of the complexity of healthcare" to one in which everyone in the organization is aligned to "declare war on error and waste" and enjoy the significant throughput improvement and cost recovery as a benefit.

These three tasks—strategy alignment, applied learning, and culture or belief system transformation—are nondelegable roles of senior leadership.

Concludes Lowell Kruse, once this strategic foundation is laid, the CEO can invest in coaching executive team members and enjoy observing the entire organization's delight in seamlessly achieving quantum results. "It is truly a pleasure to conduct my coaching rounds throughout the hospital and see the joy of each staff member as they explain with pride their most recent accomplishments. This can only become possible when the executive team establishes a flawless foundation in which staff can do their best. It cannot occur by accident."

 Kruse, after attending a Lean-Six Sigma conference presumably aimed at CEOs, remarked that all of the speakers merely described their projects. None articulated any underlying strategy. In all our research, we found only a handful of senior leaders who truly discussed the strategic aims behind their entire Lean-Six Sigma efforts. When asked to describe it, most immediately began by stating, "Let me tell you about a few of our projects."

Another way to make this point is to recall how many times you have heard someone ask, "Are you *doing* Six Sigma?" Often the response is something like, "Oh, yes! We have over 30 Black Belts and have completed more than 100 projects." Jack Welch, who popularized Six Sigma in manufacturing, would likely be horrified by this exchange. Rather, if the organization approached Lean-Six Sigma strategically, one would expect to hear, "Are you *pursuing* Six Sigma?" And an appropriate response might be, "Oh, yes, we have been pursuing Six Sigma goals in 10 strategic business processes for over three years. Our benchmark process, emergency department, has seen outlier length of stay driven to Four Sigma, or less than 1%, and fully expects Six Sigma by year-end." Note that in this second observation there is not one mention of a project. That is because to achieve this level of strategic results, a successful executive would not be able, nor see the need, to know the number of projects that have been completed. Projects, while obviously necessary to achieve results, are irrelevant. What is relevant is progress toward a strategic outcome.

This is one of the primary reasons why Lean-Six Sigma deployment can quickly fall into disfavor with the senior leadership of a healthcare organization. Senior leaders should not envision their role as selecting staff to run projects or chartering projects. Rather, they see their role, and right-fully so, as architects of strategy determination and strategy deployment. They anguish over questions such as:

- "Have we read our market and customer needs adequately?"

- "Have we set the right stretch goals and balanced them appropriately for quality, patient safety, patient satisfaction, and productivity?"

- "Are our managers executing fast enough to achieve our stretch goals?"

- "Will our current culture and belief system sustain the gains we are making?"

- "When we do falter, are we adjusting quickly enough to close the gaps?"

These are the questions that trouble senior leaders and, hence, form the foundational purpose of successful Lean-Six Sigma steering committees (or whatever the executive team calls itself). Of course, someone must attend to getting projects off the ground and growing resources, but this role most appropriately falls to staff or a Lean-Six Sigma Resource Group.

SO, WHAT IS LEAN-SIX SIGMA?

Lean-Six Sigma can be thought of as four distinct but interrelated charac-teristics (Caldwell 2004b):

- A strategy deployment approach

- A belief system

- A statistical calculation

- A suite of project improvement methods

These four characteristics are described in the following sections.

LEAN-SIX SIGMA AS A STRATEGIC DEPLOYMENT APPROACH

The presence of a strategic foundation for Lean-Six Sigma is signaled by several factors in a healthcare organization.

Strategy Deployment

Senior leaders in an organization with strategic deployment catalog their three-year and one-year stretch goals for quality, patient safety, patient satisfaction, and productivity, which are tied to the organization's strategic plan; these form the Lean-Six Sigma project selection matrix. When reading selected Lean-Six Sigma project charters (see Appendix B), a clear line of sight to the three-year and one-year goals is evident, rather than a haphazard, department-level chartering process based on short-term, nonstrategic goals.

Success is visible in an organization where Lean-Six Sigma is strategically deployed. Progress can be visualized because there is a process to measure it by using a measurement tool, such as a balanced scorecard.

Senior leaders and directors have both the responsibility and the accountability for deploying and overseeing progress in each strategic measure. An organizationwide system map illustrates the relationship between all major entities and core processes. The system map is critical in a Lean-Six Sigma approach, in part because three major areas for cost recovery in Lean-Six Sigma are the improvement of flow or throughput, the reduction of redundancies, and the reduction of Cost of Quality across the organization.

The CEO and other senior leaders on the steering committee willingly remain engaged after the initial six-month honeymoon period when a Lean-Six Sigma effort is strategically deployed. Many leading Lean-Six Sigma books and articles refer to the role of senior executives in the selection of projects and Black Belt facilitators. Such an approach is the kiss of death for executive engagement.

JCAHO Patient Throughput Standards Impact Senior Leader Roles

The Joint Commission on Accreditation of Healthcare Organizations (JCAHO) requires organizations to assess the impact of patient throughput and flow and to take action when data indicates that bottlenecks hurt the quality of care (Caldwell 2005). JCAHO initially inserted throughput standards into the accreditation process because of nationwide issues over emergency department overcrowding.

However, after several cases were analyzed, two factors became evident. First, because the ED is an entry point into the patient care continuum, many of the identified root causes of overcrowding related to interdependencies between the ED and aligned departments such as inpatient units, ancillary departments, surgery, and admissions. Therefore, the standards and survey process have evolved to include analysis of the entire patient throughput effectiveness. Fifty percent of the survey process now depends upon the tracer methodology, in which surveyors select specific patients and analyze their progression through the care continuum, using medical records, physical walk-throughs, and staff interviews. One selection criterion used by surveyors is "boarded" patients, who are being held on ED stretchers, in post-anesthesia care units (PACU), and in other holding places until they become inpatients. Further, in addition to these individual tracers, surveyors trace system issues related to medication management, infection control, evidence of the use of data in decision making, and staffing effectiveness.

Second, they realized that because throughput issues are related to systems and not to individual departments, solution requires attention at the senior leadership level. "All roads are leading to leadership and this standard aims at engaging dialogue with the leadership," said Carol Gilhooley, JCAHO's director of survey methods development (Caldwell 2005). "Many of the problems that we noticed at the 'sharp end' are that these issues are system, not functional, and, therefore, belong to leadership." Therefore, the throughput standards are housed within the Leadership section of the accreditation manual.

LEAN-SIX SIGMA AS A BELIEF SYSTEM

The second characteristic of Lean-Six Sigma—the belief system—is vital if organizations are to approach quantum levels of performance. To progress beyond simply benchmarking against others to setting a new order of performance first requires belief system transformation work at the governing board level, the executive level, and the manager level; among physician leaders; and among staff members.

Lean-Six Sigma, by definition, is virtual perfection. As such, the road to Lean-Six Sigma performance is not an endpoint, but a state of mind or a quest for quantum improvement. That is, Lean-Six Sigma performance, particularly during the first few years of strategic deployment, is a progressive set of 10-fold process improvements on the road to virtual perfection.

As Figure 1.1 illustrates, progressing from one performance plateau to the next, from below median to median to world class, requires ever-greater 10-fold improvements.

Progressing from below-median or median to top-quartile performance might be achieved with the current organizational belief system. Except in rare instances, however, driving beyond top-quartile performance to Lean-Six Sigma performance requires a radical transformation of the organizational belief system. No paradigm is a sacred cow, no bias beyond scrutiny.

A way to think about belief systems is to understand the organizational mythology. Probe staff and leaders for "the way things are done around here." Observe the behaviors of the formal and informal opinion leaders and

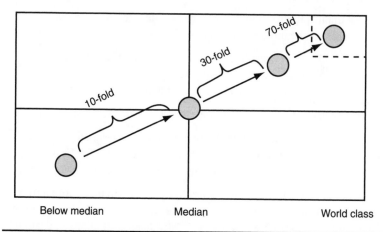

Figure 1.1   10-fold improvements to world class.

look for the kinds of advice provided by the formal and informal opinion leaders to staff facing problems or criticism.

These observations describe the organizational belief system. Once the observations are identified, the work of articulating the belief system necessary to achieve Lean-Six Sigma performance and the belief transformation exercises to close identified gaps can be undertaken.

For example, a current organizational belief system analysis might produce the following observations:

- "Healthcare is a high-hazard endeavor and errors are an unavoidable by-product of care."

- "Don't listen to what they tell you. Never, ever report an error because you will be blamed."

- "Care protocols must be at the discretion of each individual physician and nurse."

- "Regardless of what you hear, budget as low as possible because failure to achieve goals is punished here."

- "We are as good as we can be."

- "Inspect, check, and recheck constantly. It is the only way to ensure quality."

- "High quality always costs more."

As leaders begin to process the organizational belief system necessary to drive quantum improvement, the following might emerge as the observations:

- "Errors are unacceptable, and we must declare war on errors."

- "In this organization we consider it a duty to report errors and assist in the removal of all errors."

- "Unlike other organizations where you might have worked, care protocols here are always based on evidence-based medicine, and we insist on management by fact, not anecdote."

- "Status quo is never an option. Change is part of everyday work."

- "Inspection and Cost of Quality are never an assurance of high quality; it is a surrender to poor quality. We strive for Lean-Six Sigma performance in which no inspection is necessary."

Contrary to some thinking, belief systems can be transformed. In fact, belief system analysis and transformation work should always precede deployment of Lean-Six Sigma methods, teams, training, and strategy deployment. Without an underlying belief system that supports quantum improvement, aggressive process change will always be undermined, regardless of how good the Lean-Six Sigma method is. An exercise in electronic form to begin the Lean-Six Sigma belief system transformation can be found on the CD or website.

LEAN-SIX SIGMA AS A STATISTICAL CALCULATION

As a statistical calculation, Lean-Six Sigma has profound implications for understanding the relationship between quality and costs. First, as discovered by the American automobile industry in the 1980s and 1990s, errors represent the largest component of the cost of producing manufactured goods (Breyfogle 2003, 3–10). As the early Japanese quality masters discovered, as quality improves in the form of decreased waste, cost is recovered as the exhaust (Hirano 1996, 13). This is true also in healthcare enterprises.

Organizations can categorize costs into three categories (Caldwell 2004b):

- *Process cost*—The cost to run a single iteration of a process, such as producing an x-ray, performing a surgery, or caring for a patient with acute myocardial infarction. Process cost consumes approximately 67% of the total cost of a process.

- *Cost of Quality (COQ)*—The cost incurred to ensure that quality is maintained at an acceptable level. Typically, every process includes several steps, such as inspection, to make sure that the process performs as we intend.

For example, nurses check, and then recheck, to ensure that the medication they are preparing to administer to patients will not result in an allergic reaction. Case managers invest up to 90% of their time inspecting care to ensure that care paths follow protocol. All of these steps, and their underlying costs, are COQ investments. They add no value to the direct care of patients but are present to ensure quality. COQ typically consumes about 13% of the total cost, or $13 million for every $100 million in operating expense.

- *Cost of Poor Quality (COPQ)*—The cost incurred to correct processes that fail to perform as intended. Almost all processes contain some rework, work-arounds, and unexplained redundancy, not to mention the cost of malpractice and risk management. COPQ consumes approximately 20% of the total cost, or $20 million for every $100 million in operating expense.

Engineers categorize COQ and COPQ into four categories: internal failure, external failure, appraisal costs, and prevention costs (Rust 1994). As we calculate COQ and COPQ, our cost structure consumes about 33%. For example, a Louisiana medical center nursing executive calculated the number of full-time equivalent (FTE) nurses engaged in COQ and COPQ activities and determined that more than 18% of staff time was invested in tasks caused by low-quality processes. This is why Lean-Six Sigma programs are one of the most powerful tools in solving the nursing shortage.

Another organization calculated that its revenue cycle performed at less than One Sigma, consuming over 21 FTEs in COQ and COPQ alone! That is, bills that did not require manual intervention were only 7%, or much less than One Sigma, and these manual processes required 21 FTEs to process them.

So, how does Lean-Six Sigma relate quality to costs? Table 1.1 illustrates that as quality increases, COQ and COPQ decrease (Caldwell 2004b and Pande 2000, 29).

Table 1.1   Sigma levels/COQ table.

Sigma level	Defects per million opportunities (DPMO)	Quality yield	COQ/COPQ cost percent total
2	308,537	69%	Uncompetitive
3	66,807	93.3%	25–40%
4	6210	99.4%	15–25%
5	233	99.98%	5–15%
6	3.4	99.9997%	World class

As quality approaches virtual perfection—99.9997% quality yield or 3.4 errors/variations per million opportunities—COQ/COPQ nears zero. That is, if all of our first-dose antibiotics are administered in less than two hours, if all of our hip replacement patients ambulate on the first post-op day, if all AMI patients receive beta blockers within 24 hours, we have no FTEs devoted to inspecting these processes. And, there is no cost associated with rework as a result of performing the task incorrectly the first time. In other words, if our quality approaches Six Sigma levels, our avoidable costs are reduced dramatically.

LEAN-SIX SIGMA AS A SUITE OF PROJECT METHODOLOGIES

Before introducing a new methodology, executive leadership must answer two questions:

- Exactly what results are desired from the new method?

- How does this method fit in with existing methods?

These are questions related to strategically deploying Lean-Six Sigma methods, and answering them is a nondelegable role of senior leadership.

The road to fully optimizing Lean-Six Sigma improvement methods contains specific steps, which will be reviewed in Chapter 3. For now, here is a brief look at four improvement methods that can be classified within the Lean-Six Sigma framework:

- *DMAIC*—The main workhorse of all four Lean-Six Sigma methods. DMAIC is an acronym that stands for define-measure-analyze-improve-control (Pande 2000). DMAIC can be thought of as "performance improvement on steroids." While the underlying quality improvement logic of DMAIC remains similar to performance improvement methods, a significant number of tools are added to the tool bag. Typically, DMAIC is the appropriate method of choice when you believe a 10-fold process improvement potential exists, with at least $300,000 cost recovery potential (dropping to $150,000 after the first year of DMAIC use).

- *PDCA*—A traditional problem-solving approach. The logic of plan-do-check-act (Langley 1996, 6–8) as a problem-solving approach for managers has not been bested in more than 70 years. PDCA is a diagnostic-remedial process familiar to clinicians applied to management thinking, or as some have stated, "management-by-fact." PDCA is the best choice if you anticipate only a 25% process improvement with $100,000 cost recovery.

Early PDCA-type methods were tried and often abandoned because of the burdensome approach most of us took to PDCA deployment. We would strive more to ensure that everyone had a flowchart, a cause-and-effect diagram, and a Pareto chart than to achieve the critical result. In the end, managers resisted this early approach to management problem solving because too often each tool was not necessary to achieve the strategic result. PDCA used in Lean-Six Sigma deployment changes that.

Many organizations benefit from an assessment of effectiveness and impact of current methods, either before Lean-Six Sigma introduction or to increase the power of current Lean-Six Sigma and PDCA-type methods. An assessment template is available on the CD for those desiring to establish a baseline.

- *100-Day Workout*—An invigorating, execution-driven process in which process interventions begin immediately, not after a protracted period. The Workout method, built by GE upon lessons of GM's PICOs method of rapid-cycle improvement, is one of the most powerful approaches to implement minor changes that cumulatively produce major results (Breyfogle 2003, 968). The 100-Day Workout session template is scheduled to last 3½ to 4½ days, but it can be stretched into four meetings over two weeks if required. However, any period greater than two weeks reclassifies the 100-Day Workout as a manager project, having lost the critical characteristics of speed and execution orientation of 100-Day Workout.

  While perhaps not the most sophisticated method, the effectively deployed 100-Day Workout, when compared to other methods, will require the greatest transformation among managers about the best way to manage the organization. It is the best choice when the organization already possesses a workable solution set and anticipates a 5% to 15% process improvement with a $75,000 cost recovery. An example of the 100-Day Workout agenda can be found in Appendix A, in electronic versions on the CD, and at www.chipcaldwellassoc.com.

- *Manager project*—A catchall for those projects that do not fit the criteria for DMAIC, PDCA, or 100-Day Workout. Lean-Six Sigma organizations strengthen their manager project methods when they add a standardized, disciplined project management process and format. Disciplined adherence to the use of Microsoft Project, or similar project management software, along with project management training and coaching, can only accelerate the magnitude of improvements made by managers.

These concepts, over and over again, executed with diligence and without distraction, have enabled senior leaders to raise the performance bar yet another notch or two on the way to world-class levels.

CHECKLISTS AND TOOLS ACCESSIBLE ELECTROINCALLY

- DMAIC Charter—see Appendices and the CD.

- Balanced Scorecard for Lean-Six Sigma—see Chapter 4, "The Role of the Senior Leader: Achieving the Strategic Magic Moment," and the CD.

- Belief System Transformation Session Sample Agenda (with facilitator instructions)—see the CD.

- PDCA Method Assessment Template—see the CD.

- 100-Day Workout agenda—see the CD.

RECOMMENDED LEARNING SESSIONS

Learning Session for a One-Hour Senior Leader Meeting (also on CD)

One member of the executive team should serve as the recorder, capturing feedback on a flipchart.

1. Each executive takes five minutes to list the following:

   a. List three to five (but no more than five) ways that our current method of selecting and implementing projects focuses on a sequence of projects aimed at achieving a one- to three-year strategic goal that is being measured over time by a responsible executive (that is, it is strategic).

   b. List three to five (but no more than five) ways that our current method is project-by-project with only a project goal and not a long-term goal (that is, it is tactical).

2. Record responses from both lists on separate flipcharts.

3. What, if anything, can be done to ensure that the strategic factors are used more widely across the organization?

4. What, if anything, can be done to elevate the more project-by-project/tactical examples to a more strategic application?

5. Who should act upon the improvement ideas discussed? (The recorder or another accountable executive team member should be asked to capture this action plan.)

6. Set aside an hour every one to three months to review the action plan for progress.

REFERENCES

Breyfogle, Forrest. 2003. *Implementing Six Sigma,* 2nd edition. Hoboken, NJ: John Wiley & Sons.

Caldwell, Chip. 2005. Interview with Carol Gilhooley, JCAHO Director, Survey Methods Development, February 4, 2005.

Caldwell, Chip. 2004. Interview with Lowell Kruse, CEO, Heartland Health, March 24, 2004.

Caldwell, Chip, and James Brexler. 2004. "Improving Throughput and Costs Using Lean-Six Sigma." Conference presented for American College of Healthcare Executives, Key West, FL, January 12–13, 2004.

Hirano, Hiroyuki. 1996. *5S for Operators.* Portland, OR: Productivity Press.

Langley, Gerald, Kevin Nolan, Thomas Nolan, Clifford Norman, and Lloyd Provost. 1996. *The Improvement Guide.* San Francisco: Jossey-Bass Publishers.

Pande, Peter, Robert Neuman, and Roland Cavanagh. 2000. *The Six Sigma Way.* New York: McGraw Hill, 37–40.

Rust, Roland, Anthony Zahorik, and Timothy Keiningham. 1994. *Return on Quality.* Chicago: Probus Publishing.

2

The Role of Senior Leaders: Coaching Cost of Quality Recovery

We never have enough time to do it right,
but we always have enough time to do it over.

Jack Barrett, MD

"Executive leaders must be able to *coach* in the actual methods of care," observed Don Berwick, MD, president, Institute for Healthcare Improvement, during one of his popular keynote addresses at the institute's annual meetings (Berwick 1996). He goes on to advise, "We have talked about why we should improve and we have talked about where we can improve. We know scientifically where improvements can be made. . . . [Now] we need to talk about *how* we can improve." A major, nondelegable role of senior leaders is to support redesign to fully optimize Lean-Six Sigma as a strategy deployment vehicle. To coach managers and other key stakeholders in Lean-Six Sigma, leaders must be prepared to lead a dialogue in the following areas:

- Lean-Six Sigma as a cost recovery concept

- The seven categories of waste that should be known by every executive and manager

- The effect of Lean Thinking on throughput and cost recovery

- The eight Lean-Six Sigma change concepts that all executives can use to coach managers

Unlike CQI or total quality management (TQM), in which facilitators were extremely shy about cost and cost recovery in front of managers, nurses, physicians, and other key stakeholders, a key tenet of Lean-Six Sigma at the outset is the importance of stripping out process waste and Cost of Quality in all its forms. This factor is so foundational, in fact, that every project charter includes sections describing the business impact, the relationship to the organization's strategic objectives, and the potential cost recovery expected as a result of project execution. (Refer to Appendix B, CD, or website for a DMAIC charter example.) If the project charter is fully complete, an attempt to quantify cost recovery is mandatory. It is the Lean-Six Sigma Black Belt's role to ensure that cost recovery theories and linkages are fully explored, documented, and signed by the project leader and the executive champion before the project is launched. A Black Belt, a role to be discussed more fully in a Chapter 4, is a highly trained and apprenticed individual dedicated to the project manager and senior executive champion to aid in statistical, process engineering, and implementation methods; the Lean-Six Sigma Resource Group, the department in which Black Belts are housed, is charged to provide at least a 5:1 return on its expenses (Caldwell 2004a).

Cost recovery in a Lean-Six Sigma sense far exceeds the less sophisticated cost approaches found in traditional cost reduction activities and slash-and-burn consulting firms in which managers are expected to extract costs without process knowledge coaching. Lean-Six Sigma provides resources, coaching, and training in methods of process waste identification, waste removal techniques, throughput and flow improvement techniques, and methods to measure cost recovery.

 However, it remains a nondelegable role of senior leaders, as project champions and as strategy deployment agents within the organization, to establish and oversee the line-of-sight relationship between process improvement goals established for project charters and the degree of cost recovery expected. Further, it is senior leaders, not Black Belts alone, who must coach with methods of process improvement that lead to cost recovery at the exhaust of such improvements. To carry out this vital task, senior leaders must develop an expanded knowledge base and vocabulary. This knowledge base begins with an understanding of lean thinking and Six Sigma's focus on process.

HOW CAN LEAN-SIX SIGMA SERVE AS A COST RECOVERY CONCEPT?

Before understanding the relationship between process performance and process resource consumption, it is vital to understand what Six Sigma has to say about the impact of process variation. Most measures in healthcare enterprises focus on the average and provide no information about variation around the average. For example, we measure cash generation in the form of average days in accounts receivable. We measure average length of stay and we measure average cost per department. Often, we even trend these data over time, most of the time without fully understanding why our performance rises and falls month to month. One organization's length of stay might exhibit a very tight range from patient to patient, but another organization might experience wild swings in length of stay from patient to patient. Unfortunately, our reliance on managing based upon these averages provides us no knowledge of this variation nor of its influence on quality or cost. This variation produces unnecessary cost more than the average cost of the process.

 But, as one of our statistics mentors often remarked, "Focusing on the average is a bit like having one foot in hot water and one foot in ice water and observing that, on average, we feel pretty comfortable." And, as it turns out, knowledge of this variation is much more important than the temperature of the water.

As Figure 2.1 suggests, every process possesses some degree of variation. It is first important to know two pieces of information about a process: customer expectations and the capabilities of the process to meet customer expectations.

Customer Expectations

To manage Cost of Quality, the first prerequisite is to catalog expectations of customers of the process (Rust 1994). What do our customers expect of this process? For customers of an emergency department, for example, do they desire to receive care in less than four hours? Less than three hours? Note that the customer's expression of need is not in terms of the average length of stay (LOS), but rather the longest length of time. Or, for customers of the inpatient food service, do our patients expect lunch no earlier than 11:30 and no later than 12:30, or do they expect lunch no earlier

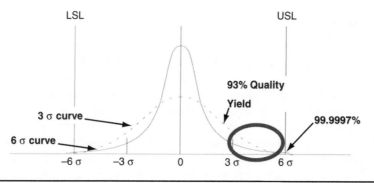

Figure 2.1   Three Sigma and Six Sigma performance curves.

than 11:45 and no later than 12:15? These customer expectations are expressed using an engineering term called upper specification limits (USL) and lower specification limits (LSL) (Pande 2000, 26–30). Figure 2.1 highlights these concepts in graphic format. The USL is designated by the circle pinpointing the customers' expectations.

Customer expectations of some processes have only an upper boundary, like ED LOS. Patients are delighted the faster we provide all necessary treatment and get them on their way, but they become annoyed beyond a certain toleration point.

Customer expectations of some processes have only a lower boundary, like time spent by the attending physician with the patient and family during rounds. Less time at a defined LSL drives perceived poor care.

Can you think of processes in which there is a USL, but not an LSL? What about an LSL, but no USL? Can you think of processes in which customers possess both a USL and an LSL?

It is possible to understand the cost recovery of a process only by detecting the USL and LSL. Most frequently, customers are not unhappy or angry about their care at the average. Ever hear ED patients complain about their ED LOS when they were treated in your *average* length of time? Not very often. Patients begin complaining at the USL—that point in time when their expectations have failed to be achieved. It also turns out that this is where our controllable costs occur. At the USL, quality has deteriorated due to poor quality, at the hands of inaccurate information; misplaced samples, medications, or information; or excessive delays caused by swings in demand. The circle in Figure 2.1 indicates where quality fails and uncessary cost and process waste begins. All of these poor quality occurrences consume resources and cost us money in the form of waste. And none of these costs add to quality, but rather detract from quality in the form of slower treatment, additional needle sticks, and so forth. Therefore, knowledge of customers' expectations is a critical first step in recovering Cost of Quality.

Process Capabilities

Knowledge of customer expectations provides us with no clue as to how often we meet their expectations. The next piece of information we require is to understand, under the best of circumstances, what is the best this process can perform? This knowledge gives clues to us about the capability of this process to achieve specific performance. If Figure 2.1 represented an emergency department, for example, we would learn whether the ED can ever produce an LOS of less than one hour and we would learn the percentage of time that LOS exceeds four hours. Of course, Lean-Six Sigma Black Belts also have a name for process capability; it is designated the upper control limit (UCL) and lower control limit (LCL). Combined with customer expectations in the form of USL and/or LSL, these boundaries, in essence, inform us of the probability that the process can achieve customer needs and for what percentage of the time.

On these two pieces of knowledge—customer expectations and process capabilities—hang all of our efforts to drive quality upward while achieving cost recovery as the exhaust of improvement efforts.

And yet, even if individual processes meet internal customer requirements, consolidated healthcare processes can fail miserably when viewed through the eyes of patients and other external customers. Consider, as an example, any four-step process owned by four different departments, such as the one shown in Figure 2.2. Assume that each department achieves a laudable 93% quality performance during the year; indeed, in many organizations, such an accomplishment might get the highest of awards at the annual quality awards meeting.

Notice, as contained in Figure 2.2, the view of this four-step process from the patients' perspective. Fewer than 75% of patients are receiving quality care. The cumulative effect in multifunctional processes, which represent a majority in healthcare, suggests unhappy patients, time after time.

Imagine the same four-step process, as highlighted in Figure 2.3, if a Lean-Six Sigma approach were taken so that each process achieves Six Sigma levels of performance.

In the case of our Lean-Six Sigma organization, the patient experiences quality 99.99% of the time. This is the process performance case for Lean-Six Sigma.

The impact of this variation in process performance most often is hidden from the organization's leadership. While complaints are the clearest signal of poor process alignment, we often seek to uncover these sources of complaints through our patient satisfaction or physician satisfaction survey process, complaints analysis, or other nonprocess knowledge discovery tools. These hidden Cost of Quality process relationships are more profound across interdependent process boundaries than internal functional process boundaries, but they exist wherever we look. Martin Miller, a consultant with Business Prototyping, Inc., through a hypothetical four-step emergency department length-of-stay simulation, simulated over a 50-week run, uncovered the relationships revealed in Table 2.1 (Caldwell 2004a).

Note that even with an increase of 33% in staffing, no improvement was achieved in the overall LOS. This is because, although service at the location of the additional FTE allocation improved dramatically, ED patients simply moved to the next bottleneck and were there stuck in a queue. How often do we respond to quality issues by throwing resources at them without fully analyzing the negative impact of throughput and bottlenecks?

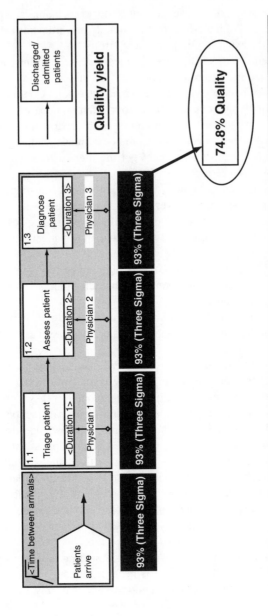

Figure 2.2　Overall quality at Three Sigma process performance.

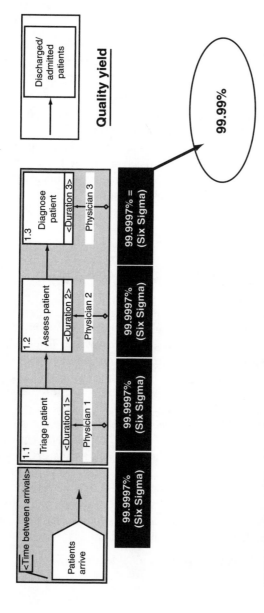

Figure 2.3   Overall quality at Six Sigma process performance.

Table 2.1   Impact of improving flow versus adding staff on process performance.

LOS	Actual	33 percent increase in staff	20 percent reduction in throughput
Low	210	210	38
Mean	260	260	45
High	310	310	53

Many of these issues can be uncovered through the system mapping encouraged in Chapter 4 and through Lean-Six Sigma simulation.

In short, flow and throughput issues are most often hidden from discovery but, through aggressive Lean-Six Sigma innovations, can dramatically improve the patient's experience, leading to improved patient satisfaction scores and recovery of Cost of Quality as exhaust.

COACHING THE SEVEN CATEGORIES OF WASTE

As a pioneer, Womack (1990) noted that before addressing process waste, the typical Toyota plant devoted 20% of its physical plant and 25% of its worked hours to waste. After addressing process waste, Toyota ultimately decreased the worked hours per car from 31 to 16, almost a 100% increase in productivity. To drive toward these levels of quality, senior leaders find it necessary to coach managers in uncovering process waste—the waste that occurs when we fail to achieve the USL or LSL. Process engineers have found it helpful to attach labels to the types of waste. Before delving into examples of waste, however, it is important to point out that engineers developed these categories, not as a means to judge managers or organizations but rather as a way to learn where waste exists and to root it out systemically. There is no useful place for judgment in these discoveries, only curiosity and open-mindedness, followed by a willingness to experiment with new processes to eliminate waste as it is found. These categories of waste, to be reviewed in detail after this listing, are as follows:

- Overproduction/overcapacity/staffing-demand variances

- Correction

- Processing

- Inventory

- Waiting

- Motion

- Material and information movement

Overproduction/Overcapacity/ Staffing-Demand Variances

The most common type of waste in healthcare organizations is providing more resources than required for the demand being placed on the process. The presence of overproduction is not always intuitive. For example, every nursing unit maintains a staffing plan that has been determined to represent nursing's definition of quality. In one Illinois medical center, the nursing division defined quality staffing on one medical-surgical unit for the 3–11 P.M. shift, when the census was 50 patients, at eight registered nurses, four patient care technicians, and two licensed practical nurses. It was the intention of the organization that as the unit census decreased, staffing would decrease accordingly. However, it was discovered that staffing coordinators were quick to add staff as census increased, but not as fast to decrease staff as the census declined. Once again, it is important to restate that these staffing levels were determined by the nursing division as quality staffing at the threshold census levels. The unit was at its most productive at 50 patients or 26 patients, with 7.84 worked hours per patient day and $119 per patient day, and at its lowest productivity at census levels of 42, 37, and 36, with worked hours per patient day of 9.3 and a cost per patient day of $138. By definition, then, the unit was in an overproduction state any time its census level was not 50 or 26 and in an extreme overproduction state any time its census level was 42, 37, or 36. Another example of overproduction would be any time a surgery suite is staffed and ready to receive a surgery patient but surgery or active prep for surgery is not under way. In the average surgery department, pure productive time, as measured by "cut-close hours" divided by staffed hourse, rarely tops 50%, or 1.5 Sigma. Every department has times and forms of overproduction.

"In Quality" versus "Out of Quality" Staffing

An important training point by senior leaders to managers at this juncture is to ask, what might we do when census drops to, say, 47? Occasionally, a manager might say, "The nurses will be able to do other things that are important." The appropriate senior leader coaching point might be, "First, aren't these staffing levels based on a high quality of care at each census level and, therefore, since it is nursing's definition of quality, shouldn't staffing decrease accordingly?" Often, a manager will respond, "Yes, but we would then be able to accept patients holding in the ED," to which a senior leader should respond, "So, then as the number of patients holding in the ED decreases, their staffing would decrease because they have fewer patients receiving care." This dialogue might continue for some time until an endpoint is agreed upon that, at some department, as patient care demands decrease, overproduction must be eliminated through a reduction in staff or an increase of new patients.

 Another effective manager skill-building approach for building understanding and application of overproduction is to conduct a meeting breakout dialogue on each manager's definition of "quality staffing" and the impact of being "in quality" or "out of quality." To effectively transform managers' thinking regarding quality staffing, a specific sequence works best, as suggested at the end of this chapter in "Learning Session for a One-Hour Director/Manager Meeting—Defining 'In Quality'/'Out of Quality' Staffing." In a meeting session or over two to three months in a structured action agenda like the 100-Day Waste Workout to recover $1 million or more in Cost of Quality, the sequence of learning lessons follows this sequence (an electronic version of this exercise, plus accompanying slides, can be accessed on the CD to guide you in conducting a learning session for managers):

1. First, and most important, as with all improvements based on reduction of waste, managers must understand that our mandate as a quality organization is to ensure that we are always seeking to be "In Quality" and never accepting of an "Out of Quality" state. During any "Out of Quality" event, very important customer needs fail to be achieved and the most important role for everyone in the organization is to ensure "Quality." It will be important for senior leaders to reiterate this notion of "In Quality" and "Out of Quality" over and over and over. You can never state it too frequently because, without exception, one or more managers will define the quest to drive out waste as a reduction in quality.

For our purposes during this advanced discussion of the category of waste called overproduction, "In Quality" and "Out of Quality" hold specific meanings. Managers must determine, based on care requirements or support requirements, depending upon their departments' function, exactly how they define *quality* in terms of the number of work units per staff person or unit. That is, for an emergency department, the nurse manager must clearly define that each nurse should average four patients at any given time, but never more than six and never fewer than three. For a medical/surgical unit, as discussed earlier, the unit manager must clearly define that, when census is at 30, five nurses should be on duty, but we should never have more than 33 patients and we should never have fewer than 27 patients. During any of these outside occurrences, we would determine that we are in an "Out of Quality Staffing" situation. The "In Quality" determination should be made hour by hour, seeking to determine the percentage of times we are "In Quality." An expected range for most functional areas is between 60% and 75%, or about Two Sigma (from Table 1.1 in Chapter 1). Therefore, if senior leaders were to set a long-term Magic Moment strategic goal of 85% minimum during any given pay period, a concept that will be discussed in great detail in Chapter 4, it is not difficult to comprehend that millions in Cost of Quality recovery would result. This is best for quality, patient safety, and efficiency. All customers win when we seek to drive out waste.

Figure 2.4 (also included in the suggested learning session slides on the CD and website) provides a good mental image of the concept of "In Quality" and "Out of Quality." This graph provides information, from "Day 1," "Day 2," "Day 3," and so on through the pay period, of the number of patients assigned to a medical/surgical unit.

2. There are times during the day that we find ourselves in an "Out of Quality" situation. One of these situations involves more demand (that is, more patients) than our current "Quality Staffing" requires and we are thus "Out of Quality" on the high end of patients per staff or unit, as illustrated in Figure 2.5. This graph provides information on the days during the pay period of how many times we achieve our "Quality Staffing" plan on a medical/surgical unit. During these times, we have too much demand or too few staff based on our definition of "Quality Staffing."

3. There are also times during the day that we find ourselves "Out of Quality" in the other direction. These situations involve less demand per staff or more staff than the demand warrants based on our definition of "Quality Staffing" (that is, fewer patients or too many staff for the demand). During these situations we are "Out of Quality" on the low end of work units per staff or unit, as shown in Figure 2.6.

When these events occur, managers should exert as much effort to get back into "Quality" as they do when they are in an "Out of Quality" state of having too much demand and hence require more staff. Alas, our experience holds that most organizations exert great effort to bring in more staff when demand exceeds "Quality Staffing," but exert very little effort when they find themselves in an "Out of Quality" situation in the opposite direction. In short, then, what senior leaders are requiring is that managers exert great effort to ensure that their functional areas remain in an "In Quality" environment for never less than 85% during any given pay period. "This is what we mean by 'Quality,'" would be an effective senior leader coaching mantra.

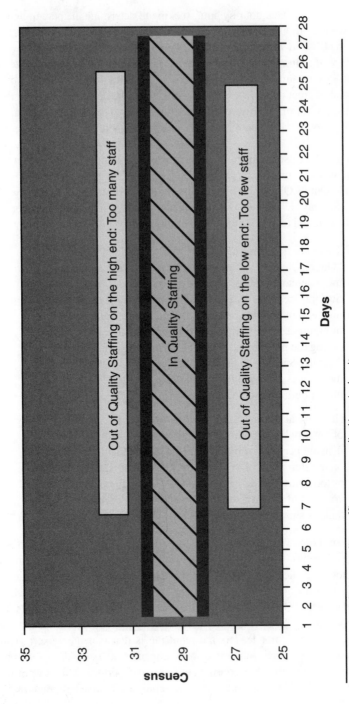

Figure 2.4   Defining quality staffing on a medical/surgical unit.

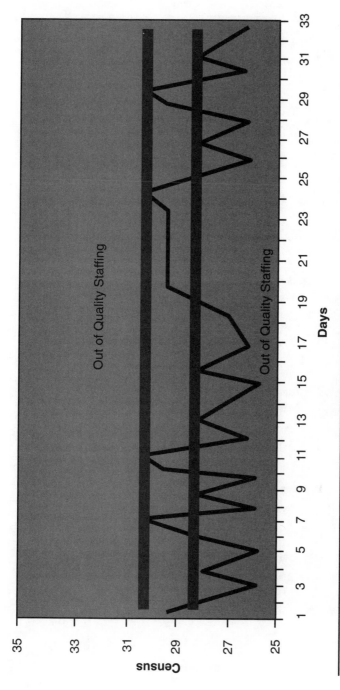

Figure 2.5   "Out of Quality" staffing—too much demand or too few staff.

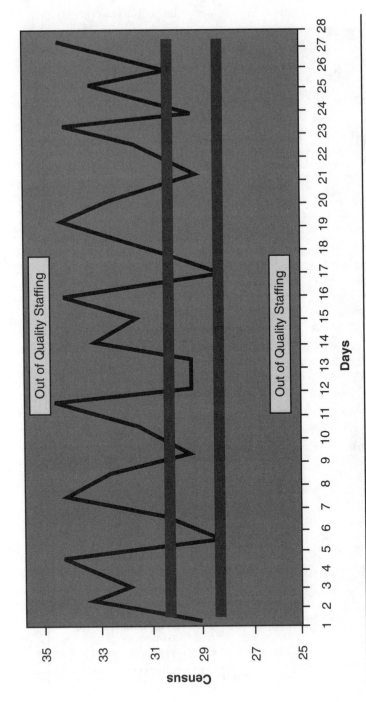

Figure 2.6 "Out of Quality" staffing—too little demand or too many staff.

4. Of course, one of our more important goals as an organization is to ensure, for every hour of the day, that we are "In Quality." This situation is shown in Figure 2.7.

To optimize this way of thinking, senior leaders begin by determining the requirements in the following categories to advance the organizations' managers to this level of enlightenment:

• Data needs

• Training needs

• Tools and support

During this process, selected senior executives can commit to implementing solutions over the next 100 days to determine the percentage of hours during the day in one or more of their departments and pilot contingency processes to increase the percentage of "In Quality" hours. These results can then be reported to the entire executive team and/or a follow-up manager meeting. An example of a manager's data collection over two pay periods is shown in Figure 2.8. Observe the number of days in which the manager is "Out of Quality" on the low end, signified by the circles, compared to the number of days the manager achieves the target.

In addition to being a recommended strategic Magic Moment, as will be discussed in Chapter 4, the "In Quality Staffing" process is an ideal follow-on 100-Day Workout, following the 100-Day Waste Workout, with the goal for each manager to individually calculate the percentage of hours during the day that they are "In Quality" and to implement changes during the 100-Day Workout to dramatically increase their "In Quality" percentage. Again, an external coach is highly effective in this type of exercise, bringing experience into the dialogue and often pushing managers' paradigms beyond the limits that internal staff can accomplish.

By far, overproduction and failure to match staffing and capacity to demand is the most far-reaching type of waste and the one that produces the most Cost of Quality recovery potential. Moreover, overproduction is fairly easy to detect compared to some of the six other types of waste.

Correction

The second type of waste is overcorrection. A state of overcorrection exists whenever an inspection, or correction, occurs. As expressed so eloquently by Don Berwick, MD, "inspection isn't an assurance of high quality, it is a surrender to poor quality" (Berwick 1996). That is, if the process were performed without deficiency in the first place, inspection and inspectors that

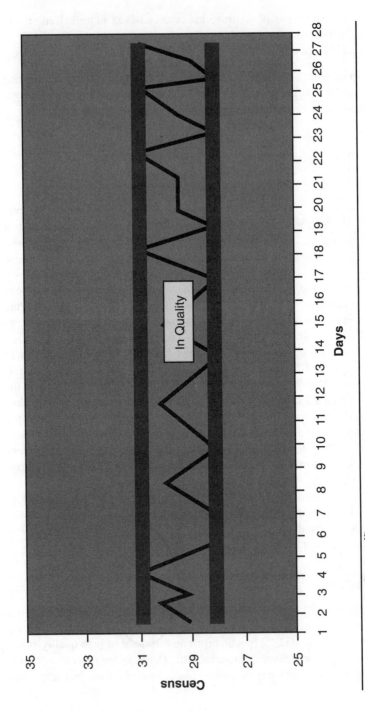

Figure 2.7 "In Quality" staffing.

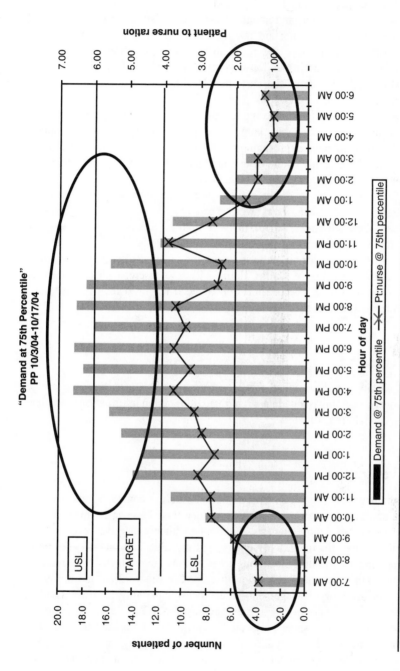

Figure 2.8 Example "In Quality" staffing assessment.

perform inspection could be deployed to other work. Every process contains some inspection and should clearly be called an enemy of quality. These inspections do not aid quality, but rather they exist only because processes contain errors and result in poor quality in the minds of customers. After all, an inspection takes time and an avoidable delay is poor quality in the minds of the customer. Healthcare organizations can spot inspection wherever they look. In some instances, entire departments are devoted to inspection. For example, case managers dedicate about 75% of their time to inspection, checking to ensure that physicians have responded to the latest diagnostic information or to ensure that the physician has written a discharge order. None of this activity adds value to patient care, but rather it slows the progress of care. If case managers were able to invest 75% of their time to direct patient care rather than to inspecting care, patients and case managers would benefit. Inspection occurs in non–patient care activities as much or more than in direct care processes. For example, in one midwestern medical center, 21 staff were devoted to inspecting claims for correctness before they were sent to payors. What is the level of quality of claims, defined as zero discrepancies on the first pass? A scant 7%. The organization reduced the need for over five staff positions as the level of quality was improved to above 70%.

Processing

Processing waste occurs whenever a process is redundant. A good example of overprocessing is a patient's reciting demographic information more than one time during a visit.

Inventory

Inventory waste is the one most recognized and, of course, occurs any time the organization maintains more inventory than its material management system par-level table suggests. A dialogue with any caregiver reveals secret hiding places for linen, wheelchairs, and the like. The necessity for these supplemental inventory locations arises because internal customer requirements—the customer expectation discussed in Figure 2.1—and the variation in inventory management—the process capability also discussed in Figure 2.1—are not in synch. Because only about 2% of a healthcare organization's balance sheet is devoted to inventory, compared to over 50% work in progress for the typical manufacturing company, just-in-time inventory is not the magic bullet in healthcare as it was for manufacturing. However, overinventory remains a minor category of waste.

Waiting

A senior vice president at a major quality think tank remarked to one author, "Healthcare is the only industry I have ever heard of that actually has a name for a major category of waste. You have waiting rooms. Most organizations outside of healthcare would go bankrupt if they thought like this." We also have functions such as the holding area in surgery, in which patients are inconveniently housed while waiting for lab results, EKG results, the surgeon, and the anesthesiologist to catch up with one another. In the patient's mind, this is poor quality. In the staff's mind, this is poor quality. And, it is a major source of Cost of Quality and Cost of Poor Quality.

Motion

Motion waste occurs, in principle, any time a patient is moved. From a purely process engineering perspective, the highest level of quality would be for the patient to be escorted to her room and all registration, intake, diagnostic tests, and therapeutic interventions to occur in this room. During times that intensive care staffing levels were required, rather than move the patient, caregiver hours would simply be increased until that intensive care was no longer required. This would be best both for quality and for cost. The major reason patients are moved from intensive care into medical-surgical care, aside from minor equipment differences in care settings, is for the management of nursing hours of care, not for quality. In fact, Mayo's Luther-Midelfort facility documented that 56% of its medication errors occurred at the "interfaces of care" (Rebillot 2000). If error events are generalized from medication errors to errors and delays of all types, it could be argued that transporting patients is a hazard to both quality and cost.

Material and Information Movement

Similar to patient movement, movement of materials and information throughout the organization is a drain on resources and quality.

HOW CAN SENIOR LEADERS
REDUCE THIS WASTE?

Grounding senior leaders, managers, and physicians regarding the negative impact of process waste on quality and the deteriorating effect on resource drainage can be one of the most powerful efforts that a healthcare organization can undertake. A popular way of imparting this knowledge is to engage managers in a "Waste Walk," a three-hour learning experience crafted by a Chip Caldwell and Associates staff member, Sherry Bright, in 2000 (Caldwell 2004a). One form of Waste Walk allots 35 points to each team, to be allocated between the seven categories of waste (Bichino 2000). Managers are oriented to the categories of waste and sent out in groups of three or four into the hospital to uncover examples of waste. Upon return, managers share their examples. An example of this form can be found in Appendix A. When combined with a 100-Day Workout devoted to operations waste reduction, the impact can be significant, in most cases returning over $1 million in Cost of Quality recovery. The 100-Day Workout methodology will be covered in detail in Chapter 3 on project methods. A three-hour Waste Walk form appears in Figure 2.9.

Key point	Observations	Ideas to eliminate	Estimated cost recovered if eliminated
Overproduction/ Overcapacity (see below stated goal level) **Staffing-to-demand** (greater than stated staffing ratio at this moment)			
Correction (inspection & rework)			
Processing			
Inventory			
Waiting			
Motion of people			
Material & information movement			

Figure 2.9   100-Day Waste Walk.

WHAT IS THE IMPACT OF LEAN THINKING ON THROUGHPUT AND COST?

Six Sigma and waste reduction by themselves fail to open up all the opportunities hidden within healthcare processes. It has been well demonstrated that Six Sigma alone can take an organization only so far (Chowdhury 2002). This is particularly true in healthcare in which flow and throughput outweighs inventory overages by a large margin. Many processes, particularly those in which throughput or flow is a major process feature, mask inefficiencies deep within themselves. A mind-set and accompanying tool set found within the discipline known as lean production is required for recovering these opportunities.

What Is Lean and How Can It Be Applied?

Experiences in other industries provide interesting insights into the roots of lean thinking. Womack (1996) recites a case study of Doyle Wilson Homebuilder of Austin, Texas, which, using lean techniques, redesigned the process of constructing a new home from six months to one month. How? The principles of lean, followed by Doyle Wilson Homebuilder and other organizations that optimize lean, are as follows (Bichino 2000):

- Focus on the value stream, that is, those process steps that add value to the customer.

- Flow, which involves three critical thinking skills, as follows:

  - Focus on the output or goal from the customers' viewpoints.

  - Ignore process boundaries and limitations of job descriptions.

  - Eliminate bottlenecks and rework.

Stalk and Hout (1990), pioneers in evolving lean thinking into practical applications, note a significant difference between traditional organizations and lean organizations, as shown in Table 2.2.

Table 2.2   Traditional organizations versus lean organizations.

Traditional Organizations	Lean Organizations
• Improve function by function	• Focus on systems, especially interfaces
• Work in departments, batch	• Generate continuous flow or throughput
• Invest to reduce cost	• Invest to reduce time

Henderson (2002) notes that for those processes in which flow is a critical characteristic, the secrets of successful eradication of process waste are:

- Specify in measurable terms the customers' needs and expectations for speed.

- Analyze the entire process, including those that support the core process, to determine the weakest links.

- Redesign processes to solve for the weakest link (then solve the next one, and so on). Level 1 Trauma Center 656-bed Inova Fairfax Medical Center (HCAB 2002) has been one of the first to illustrate the point that it is a waste of resources to solve flow issues unless the point of attack is the most impactful bottleneck (weakest link). Using lean principles, the hospital decreased inpatient bed placement from two hours to 30 minutes, resulting in the number of admissions per day increasing from 127 to 163.

- Balance the flow for optimal cycle time and resource consumption (ensuring that resources contribute to customer needs).

However, drawing upon the power of lean often demands a radical redefinition of quality and the roles of key professionals who perform care functions. Recognizing the transformational approach required to make lean effective, Goldratt (Dettmer 1997) suggested the following process:

1. Define the current state in flow chart form so that interprocess and intraprocess relationships are observable.

2. Codify the desired future state in flowchart form so that differences can be visualized.

3. Uncover conflicts between the current and desired future states and create a conflict resolution diagram.

4. Charter the transformation plan, an orderly progression from current state to desired future state, based upon the political and environmental realities.

How Can Improving Throughput Reduce Cost? Three Types of Cost Recovery

Before beginning any discussion about process throughput, process cost, and cost recovery, it might first be beneficial to review the relationships between process variables and cost. Mozena (1999) notes that "costs are not causes," but rather that they are symptoms of the interrelationships between processes. Not all process improvement opportunities will return cost recovery as the exhaust, nor will all improvements yield cost recovery without additional activity on the part of leadership. Generally, the following paradigms prove helpful in determining the additional effort required, if any, to extract cost from three types of process throughput improvements:

- *Type 1*—A process throughput improvement produces a direct cost recovery. For example, an emergency department (ED) reduction in length of stay (LOS) results in three types of savings without any additional effort on the part of leadership. First, a significant reduction in diversion minutes is likely, producing additional incremental profit with no new staffing. Second, patients leaving without treatment (LWOT) will decrease without any additional activity. Third, a Type 2 savings occurs in worked hours per ED visit.

- *Type 2*—A process throughput improvement that produces time saved but no cost recovery without an additional action to impact worked hours per unit of service. As in the previous ED example, two events will automatically occur under a Type 1 savings, requiring no action on the part of leadership, but one Type 2 savings results. This Type 2 savings is ED nurse worked hours per ED visit. As Figure 2.10 illustrates, if ED LOS averages four hours and ED worked hours per visit approach 3 hours per ED visit, then the department is investing 0.75 worked hours for every ED patient hour.

As a throughput improvement concept, lean thinking suggests that, as throughput improves, staff time is saved in the form of reduced staff worked hours per unit of service. For example, if ED LOS decreases, which is a throughput improvement, staff time is saved in the form of reduced patient care hours required of ED staff. If ED LOS decreases 25%, to three hours, as illustrated in Figure 2.11 on page 40–41, then 0.75 worked hours are freed up for every ED patient.

However, these savings are not driven automatically to the bottom line without additional activity. To capitalize on this gained economy, the organization's leadership must reduce the hours during which selected ED rooms are staffed. In other words, in a Type 2 savings, the demand curve on the ED will decrease significantly, but to recover any portion of this 0.75 worked hours per ED visit, the ED management must adjust the hours during which selected rooms are operational. It is important to note, however, that 100% of the conversion of time saved into reduced worked hours per unit of service is

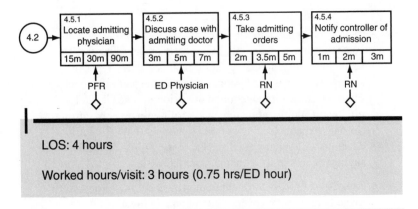

Emergency Department Process Model
Main ED
4.0 Disposition Patient
4.5 Admit Patient

LOS: 4 hours

Worked hours/visit: 3 hours (0.75 hrs/ED hour)

Figure 2.10   LOS and worked hours relationship.   *(Continued on page 39.)*

exceedingly rare. As a rule of thumb, the organization can expect to recover between at least 50% of the time saved, or, in our ED example, about $250,000, but not more than 75%, or about $300,000. As Figure 2.12 on page 42 highlights, as emergency department length of stay decreases, worked hours per ED visit decrease accordingly (Caldwell 2004a).

   Another schema to help illustrate this concept is shown in Table 2.3 on page 43. Note in the final column that, as emergency department length-of-stay decreases, staffing at each hour of the day decreases, providing a reduction of 14.9 RN worked hours per day (or over five full-time equivalent staff), capturing almost $200,000 in Cost of Quality.

Type 2 savings are the most common. In fact, almost every department, with the proper training and Black Belt support, can derive significant cases of Type 2 savings. In the case of surgery, for example, if we are able to improve surgery throughput, reducing hours per operating room case by 30 minutes, we realize cost recovery only if we are able to close selected operating rooms earlier in the day. Another example would be improving the rate

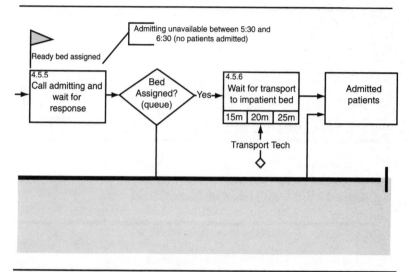

Figure 2.10   LOS and worked hours relationship.

of "noon discharge" for inpatients so that over 80% of patients leave the inpatient setting by 2 P.M., just before shift change. In this case, the 3–11 P.M. shift must be adjusted for the new evening shift patient demand. A third example would be reduced medical errors (including near misses). If nurses invest over 15% of their time inspecting and correcting medication errors and near misses, a 50% reduction in medication errors would produce at least 50% recovery of the time saved. However, converting saved nurse time into decreased worked hours is a complicated process.

- *Type 3*—A throughput savings improvement that produces optimized capacity. The underlying process throughput improvement for Type 3 savings is identical to Type 2 except that costs are recovered in the form of additional patients. In Type 2, worked hours per unit of service will decrease because staffed hours decrease. In Type 3 savings, worked hours per unit of service decrease because more patients are treated and

Emergency Department Process Model
Main ED
4.0 Disposition Patient
4.5 Admit Patient

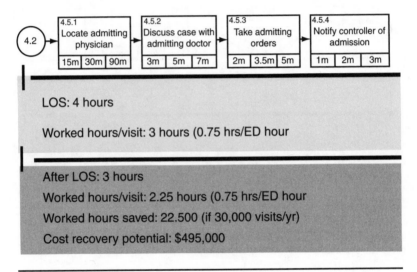

4.5.1 Locate admitting physician	**4.5.2** Discuss case with admitting doctor	**4.5.3** Take admitting orders	**4.5.4** Notify controller of admission
15m	30m	90m	3m	5m	7m	2m	3.5m	5m	1m	2m	3m

LOS: 4 hours

Worked hours/visit: 3 hours (0.75 hrs/ED hour

After LOS: 3 hours

Worked hours/visit: 2.25 hours (0.75 hrs/ED hour

Worked hours saved: 22.500 (if 30,000 visits/yr)

Cost recovery potential: $495,000

Figure 2.11   Worked hours reduced as LOS decreases.

(Continued on page 41.)

released in the same staffed time. In our previous ED example, we can convert our throughput improvement into a Type 3 savings if we can increase the number of patients treated, through either additional aggressive promotion or natural growth. In the case of surgery, for example, if we are able to improve surgery throughput, reducing hours per OR case by 30 minutes, we can capture Type 3 savings if we have surgeons willing to provide more cases because additional preferred surgery hours are available. Type 3 savings are by far the highest return on effort because we increase net revenue but incur almost no additional costs. However, Type 3 savings are less common, of course, unless the marketing department can drive additional volume or the organization's service area grows.

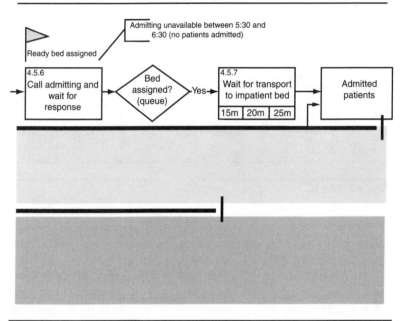

Figure 2.11 Worked hours reduced as LOS decreases.

HOW CAN WE REDUCE WORKED HOURS?

Many organizations are finding that "squeezing more blood out of the turnip" from cost center–level productivity comparative benchmarks is becoming more and more challenging. After all, the executive team and operations managers have been pursuing cost efficiencies using comparative data for a decade and, while great variation remains, creative solutions are becoming much more elusive. Establishing Lean-Six Sigma goal parameters for Types 1, 2, and 3 cost recovery is accelerated upon provision of reliable comparative cost data. One approach is to seek benchmarks from increasingly competitive marketplaces. The *LA Confidential* comparative database uses Los Angeles County, California, from Chip Caldwell

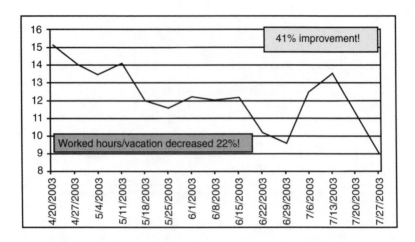

Figure 2.12   LOS improvement produces a decrease in worked hours.

& Associates (Caldwell 2004b), which is on average about 20% more aggressive than the traditional national peer grouping technique. For example, the national average for ED worked hours per unit of service from our research suggests 2.8 worked hours per ED visit, with the national top quartile at 2.1. However, the *LA Confidential* top quartile is 1.8 worked hours per unit of service (Caldwell 2004b). As found in the *Good to Great in Healthcare* research, quantum improvers seek out the most aggressive comparative benchmarks that can be found and set their goals for Lean-Six Sigma upon these rather than the less aggressive national benchmarks (Pieper 2004). The problem with this approach is that it still provides no creative solutions, only resource comparisons, and, of course, it is no substitute for the organization's existing comparative data vendor for ongoing analysis.

Great work is emerging from those Lean-Six Sigma initiatives seeking to optimize throughput, optimize capacity to demand, and/or reduce redundant processes. Readers should be careful not to limit their search for flow and capacity optimization to only the Lean-Six Sigma world. The Healthcare Advisory Board, for example, has published exception reports on emergency department and patient care throughput (Healthcare Advisory Board 2002).

However, many Lean-Six Sigma project goals recover COQ with no additional adjustments, like ED LOS, surgery first-case start times, surgery-to-follow case cycle time, and almost any dimension of patient care throughput. The projects strive to reduce total LOS or cycle times, which produce "exhaust" cost recovery.

Table 2.3 Hour-by-hour staffing savings from throughput improvement.

MHC						
		RN adjust to decreased demand				
		Current		After 14 percent improvement		
Time	Volume number points in area state of hour	Staffing (beginning of hour) RNs	Volume number points in area Points/RN	Staffing (beginning of hour) start of hour	RNs (@ same)	RN decr
700	3.1	3.6	0.9	2.6	3.1	0.5
800	3.4	3.7	0.9	2.9	3.2	0.5
900	4.0	4.4	0.9	3.4	3.8	0.6
1000	5.2	4.4	1.2	4.5	3.8	0.6
1100	7.1	4.8	1.5	6.1	4.1	0.7
1200	8.9	5.1	1.8	7.7	4.4	0.7
1300	8.8	5.2	1.7	7.6	4.5	0.7
1400	9.6	5.1	1.9	8.2	4.4	0.7
1500	10.7	5.3	2.0	9.2	4.5	0.7
1600	10.4	5.1	2.0	9.0	4.4	0.7
1700	11.9	5.6	2.1	10.2	4.9	0.8
1800	11.4	5.3	2.2	9.8	4.5	0.7
1900	12.8	5.3	2.4	11.0	4.5	0.7
2000	12.4	5.4	2.3	10.6	4.6	0.8
2000	12.7	5.4	2.4	10.9	4.6	0.8
2100	11.9	5.3	2.2	10.2	4.5	0.7
2200	10.6	4.4	2.4	9.2	3.8	0.6
2300	10.2	3.8	2.7	8.8	3.3	0.5
2400	8.6	3.5	2.4	7.4	3.0	0.5
100	6.4	3.4	1.9	5.5	2.9	0.5
200	4.1	2.9	1.4	3.6	2.5	0.4
300	3.6	2.7	1.3	3.1	2.3	0.4
400	2.9	2.5	1.2	2.5	2.2	0.4
500	2.4	2.5	1.0	2.1	2.2	0.4
600	1.1	1.4	0.8	1.0	1.2	0.2
Avg	7.8	4.2	1.7	6.7	3.7	14.9
					Hours/Yr	5424
					$/Yr	$ 189,837

EIGHT LEAN-SIX SIGMA SOLUTION SET

Tom Nolan, an international leader in quality systems, crafted 70 engineering solution suggestions from which senior leaders, managers, and quality professionals can brainstorm specific process improvement ideas (Langley 1996, 294). These broad categories, which he calls "change concepts," are not specific process improvement ideas, but rather general thought-provoking categories that can aid in shaping specific changes. For example, hip replacement demand-matching protocols, as a specific recommended change, would fall under the category of "standardization." In extending the use of the notion of change concepts in Lean-Six Sigma work, we have found it helpful to affinitize the change concepts into eight categories that simplify the task of senior manager coaching in the pursuit of process throughput and waste reduction (Caldwell 2004a). These categories, found in Figure 2.13 on pages 46–47, enable senior leaders to guide managers and other process owners in generalized approaches to improve process throughput and waste.

Taken together, these eight Lean-Six Sigma solutions can profoundly improve throughput, eliminate waste, and extract the associated Cost of Quality.

However, as noted in Rogers' work (1995), the diffusion of innovation requires attention to more factors than simply creativity. The organization must communicate the value of the innovation across multiple channels, must address the rate of adoption of change across the entire organization, and must attend to the organization and representative professional group social system norms relative to the change.

SUMMARY

It is a nondelegable role of senior leaders to coach using the new methods of improvement, and this leadership begins with understanding Six Sigma, lean thinking, cost recovery, and Lean-Six Sigma solution sets. It is only through a comprehensive understanding of these concepts that senior leaders can fully understand their roles and the roles of Black Belts and managers, and be able to manage the infrastructure necessary to drive quantum improvement and optimize the power of Lean-Six Sigma as a strategy deployment approach.

CHECKLISTS AND TOOLS ACCESSIBLE ELECTRONICALLY

- "In Quality"/"Out of Quality" Staffing Facilitation slides—see electronic version on the CD or the website, www.chipcaldwellassoc.com.

- Project Charter template—see Appendix B and the CD or website.
- Waste Walk form—see Appendix A and the electronic version on the CD.
- Lean-Six Sigma Solution Set—see appendices and the electronic version on the CD.
- Glossary—found at the end of the book and on the CD.

1. Failure modes contingency plans.

2. Consolidate functions/processes; eliminate steps.

3. Initiate dependent subprocess earlier.

4. Parallel process non-dependent processes.

5. Decrease subprocess cycle time.

6. Decrease waste, errors, waits, and delays.

7. Match staffing and capacity to demand.

8. Shape demand.

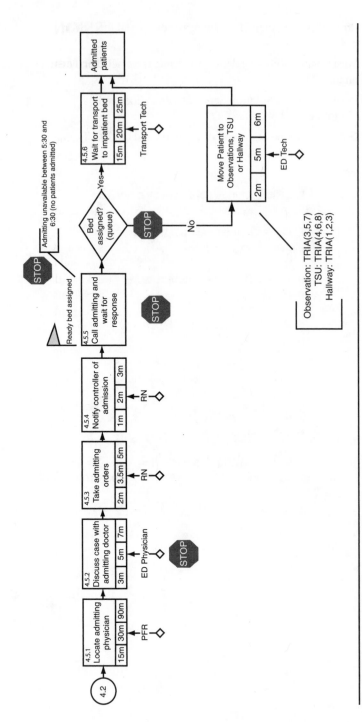

Figure 2.13 Lean-Six Sigma solution set.

Access an electronic version of the complete Lean-Six Sigma solution set on the CD or website.

RECOMMENDED LEARNING SESSIONS

Learning Session for a Two-Hour Senior Leader Meeting— Executive Waste Walk

One member of the executive team should serve as the recorder, capturing feedback on a flipchart. Alternatively, an external coach is highly effective in this type of exercise, bringing experience into the dialogue and pushing managers' paradigms beyond the limits that internal staff can accomplish. Using the Waste Walk form found in Appendix B or on the CD, the executive team should divide into groups of three (yes, including the CEO).

1. Briefly review the descriptions of the types of waste discussed in this chapter; then adjourn for a 45-minute Waste Walk.

2. During the Waste Walk, each executive team tours at least two areas of the medical center to observe waste in action and to come up with one idea for a solution on pages 2 and 3 of the Waste Walk form. Teams may record as many observations in each category as they desire, but their work is not complete until they have at least one observation in each category.

3. Upon returning, the recorder captures a few examples from each category.

4. (Optional) Using the ideas captured during this process, selected senior executives commit to implementing solutions over the next 100 days to reduce waste and/or improve throughput in their departments.

Note: This process is similar to the one followed during a 100-Day Operations Waste Workout, discussed in Chapter 3. The 100-Day Operations Waste Workout is one of the most powerful project methods for rapidly extracting Cost of Quality at the department process level.

Learning Session for a Two-Hour Director/Manager Meeting—Waste Walk

Adapt from the process above, providing a flipchart for each table of eight to ten managers.

Note: This process is similar to the one followed during a 100-Day Operations Waste Workout, discussed in Chapter 3. The 100-Day Operations Waste Workout is one of the most powerful project methods for rapidly extracting Cost of Quality at the department process level.

Learning Session for a One-Hour Director/Manager Meeting—Defining "In Quality"/"Out of Quality" Staffing

One member of the executive team or someone familiar with hospital staffing planning processes should serve as the facilitator. Alternatively, an external coach is highly effective in this type of exercise, bringing experience into the dialogue and pushing managers' paradigms beyond the limits that internal staff can accomplish. This exercise is slightly scripted to ensure that the important learning sequence is followed; however, feel free to tailor the exact phraseology to your specific communication style. Following the slides included on the CD will make this task easier.

1. Briefly orient managers to the four states of "Quality Staffing" discussed in this chapter, ideally using the slides from the CD or website, as follows:

   a. The first, and most vital, concept to express at the beginning and frequently during the dialogue, during this session, and in the weeks and months that follow, is that our mandate is to ensure that we are always seeking to be "In Quality" and never accepting of an "Out of Quality" state. During any "Out of Quality" event, very important customers' needs fail to be achieved. The most important role for everyone in the organization is to ensure "Quality."

   b. (Slide 1, "Quality Staffing") How do you define "Quality Staffing" in your area in terms of the minimum, the target or average, and the maximum number of work units per staff person or unit for each hour of the day (for example, the number of ED patients per nurse or the number of patients per medical/surgical unit)?

   c. (Slide 2, "Out of Quality") State, "There are times during the day that we find ourselves 'Out of Quality.' These situations involve more demand (more work units) than our current 'Quality Staffing' requires, and we are thus 'Out of Quality' on the high end of work units per staff or unit. When these events occur, which customers lose, and what is the impact?" Record your observations on a flipchart.

   d. (Slide 3, "Out of Quality") State, "There are times during the day that we find ourselves 'Out of Quality' in the other direction. These situations involve less demand per staff or more staff (fewer work units or too many staff for the demand) than our current 'Quality Staffing' requires, and we are thus 'Out of Quality' on the low end of work units per staff or unit. When these events occur, which customers lose, and what is the impact?" Record your observations on a flipchart.

   e. (Slide 4, "In Quality") State, "Of course, one of our more important goals as an organization is to ensure, for every hour of the day, that we are "In Quality."

2. Breakout question (the best way for all to learn) or large group discussion: State, "This is best for all customers. What might be needed for us to increase our rate of 'In Quality' hours as a percentage of the 24-hour day in each category?"

- Data

- Training

- Tools

- Support

- Other

3. (Optional) Using the ideas captured during this process, selected senior executives commit to implementing solutions over the next 100 days to determine the percentage of hours during the day in one or more of their departments and pilot contingency processes to increase the percentage of "In Quality" hours. These results can be reported at the entire executive team or at a follow-up managers meeting. An example of a manager's data collection over two pay periods can be found in the slides in "In Quality" staffing on the CD or website.

Note: This process is an ideal follow-on 100-Day Workout, following the 100-Day Waste Workout, with the goal for each of the managers to individually calculate the percentage of hours during the day that they are "In Quality" and to implement changes during the 100-Day Workout to dramatically increase their "In Quality" percentage. Again, an external coach is highly effective.

REFERENCES

Berwick, Donald. 1996. *Run to Space*. Video. Boston: Institute for Healthcare Improvement.

Bichino, John. 2000. *The Lean Toolbox*, 2nd edition. Buckingham, England: PICSIE Books, 12–13, 74–75.

Breyfogle, Forrest. 2003. *Implementing Six Sigma*, 2nd edition. Hoboken, NJ: John Wiley & Sons.

Caldwell, Chip. 2004. "Good to Great in Healthcare: A Research Initiative." Conference presented by the American College of Healthcare Executives, St. Louis, May 26, 2004.

Caldwell, Chip, and James Brexler. 2004. "Improving Throughput and Costs Using Lean–Six Sigma." Conference presented by the American College of Healthcare Executives, Key West, FL, January 12–13, 2004.

Caldwell, Chip, and Bruce Tilley. 2004. "Aggressive Cost Reduction Using Lean–Six Sigma." National teleconference presented by the VHA and the American College of Healthcare Executives, Dallas, March 25, 2004.

Chowdhury, Subir. 2002. *Design for Six Sigma*. Chicago: Dearborn Trade, 1.

Dettmer, H. William. 1997. *Goldratt's Theory of Constraints*. Milwaukee: ASQ Quality Press.

Healthcare Advisory Board. 1999. *The Clockwork ED*. Washington: Advisory Board Company.

———. 2002. *Maximizing Hospital Capacity*. Washington: Advisory Board Company.

Henderson, Bruce, and Jorge Larco. 2002. *Lean Transformation*. Richmond, VA: Daklea Press, 58–61.

Langley, Gerald, Kevin Nolan, Thomas Nolan, Clifford Norman, and Lloyd Provost. 1996. *The Improvement Guide*. San Francisco: Jossey-Bass Publishers.

Mozena, James, Charles Emerick, and Steven Black. 1999. *Stop Managing Costs*. Milwaukee: ASQ Quality Press, 17.

Pande, Peter, Robert Neuman, and Roland Cavanagh. 2000. *The Six Sigma Way*. New York: McGraw Hill.

Rebillot, K. 2000. "Tackling Medication Errors Head On." In *Reducing Medical Errors and Improving Patient Safety: Success Stories from the Front Lines of Medicine, Accelerating Change Today for America's Health*. Washington: National Coalition on Health Care and Institute for Healthcare Improvement.

Rogers, Everett. 1995. *Diffusion of Innovations*, 4th edition. New York: Free Press, 11–25.

Rust, Roland, Anthony Zahorik, and Timothy Keiningham. 1994. *Return On Quality*. Chicago: Probus Publishing.

Stalk, George, and Thomas Hout. 1990. *Competing Against Time*. New York: Free Press, 172.

Womack, James. 1990. *The Machine That Changed the World*. New York: HarperCollins, 57 and 81.

Womack, James, and Daniel Jones. 1996. *Lean Thinking*. New York: Simon & Schuster.

ADDITIONAL READING

Cost of Quality Concepts: Pande, Peter, Robert Neuman, and Roland Cavanaugh. 2000. *The Six Sigma Way.* NY: McGraw Hill. 163–181.

Caldwell, Chip, and Charles Denham. 2001. *Medication Safety and Cost Recovery.* Chicago: Health Administration Press.

Clinical Initiatives Center. 2002. *Optimizing CCU Throughput.* Washington: Advisory Board Company.

Healthcare Advisory Board. 1999. *The Clockwork ED.* Washington: Advisory Board Company.

———. 2002. *Maximizing Hospital Capacity: Expediting Patient Throughput in an Era of Shortage.* Washington: Advisory Board Company.

Nolan, Thomas, Marie W. Schall, Donald M. Berwick, and Jane Roessner. 1996. *Reducing Delays and Waiting Times.* Boston: Institute for Healthcare Improvement.

3

The Role of Senior Leaders: Organizing Lean-Six Sigma Project Methodologies to Drive Change

The major difference between rats and people is that rats learn from experience.

B. F. Skinner

Before introducing new improvement methods associated with Lean-Six Sigma into the organization, senior leaders must answer two questions:

• Exactly what results are desired from the new methods?

• How will they fit with existing improvement methods?

Because these questions are related to strategically deploying Lean-Six Sigma methods, answering them is a nondelegable role of senior leadership.

Lean-Six Sigma is more than just a project execution method. It is a strategy deployment tool (more fully explored in Chapter 4). When organizations deploy Lean-Six Sigma from a tactical, project-driven focus rather than a strategic focus, their efforts often look like unrelated, nonstrategic projects strung together. A tactical approach greatly suboptimizes the power of Lean-Six Sigma. The road to a strategically driven, fully optimized Lean-Six Sigma deployment is evidenced by the following steps:

1. Beginning with the system map discussed in detail in Chapter 4, conduct a performance assessment of the six to ten core processes that make up the enterprise.

2. Enhance the capabilities of all improvement methods and deploy new ones to fill identified gaps.

3. Create a project selection matrix, based upon the process improvement potential and Cost of Quality recovery expectations.

4. Establish processes to track projects and results, preferably using a rapid deployment approach such as the 100-Day Plan.

5. Assess strategic results and rechart the course every 100 days.

Step 5 is referred to as the 100-Day Management Method and parallels the deployment of 100-Day Workouts.

These five steps are presented here only for construct purposes and will be detailed in Chapter 4. The remaining discussion in this chapter explains the various project methods necessary to make a strategic framework explained in Chapter 4 useful.

Very often Lean-Six Sigma deployments are described as containing only one project method—DMAIC, explained below. However, thinking of Lean-Six Sigma as only one method is to categorize it as a tactical, project-driven approach, as opposed to an organizationwide strategy deployment tool. No one project method can suffice for an organization with disparate strategic goals, functions, and staff competencies.

In our strategic framework, the traditional Lean-Six Sigma deployment suite is composed of four improvement methodologies:

- DMAIC project method—An acronym for the five major steps: define, measure, analyze, improve, and control (Pyzdek 2000, 39).

- PDCA-type project method—an acronym for plan-do-check-act (Pyzdek, 37), the project approach traditionally used in healthcare for the past decade.

- 100-Day Workout—A 2½–3½-day rapid cycle implementation project method popularized by General Electric (Breyfogle 2003, 968–987; Senge 1999, 72–82; Caldwell 2004a).

- Manager project—A catchall description for strategic projects that do not fit the characteristics of the above project methods, yet still require disciplined project planning and tracking.

In our Lean-Six Sigma cost recovery consulting work, we often jokingly point to projects that exhibit characteristics of a five-project method—"wing and a prayer," because no disciplined process can be discerned.

However, from the *Good to Great in Healthcare* research (Caldwell 2004c), it is interesting to note that quantum improvers, those organizations in the top quartile of performance, all used a disciplined project approach and a disciplined implementation method, as opposed to nonstarters, those organizations in the bottom-performing quartile, which did not use a disciplined project method.

Each of these Lean-Six Sigma project methods has a specific potential for process improvement and expected Cost of Quality recovery. An organization can expect quantum improvement from each DMAIC project. When constructed using a strategic deployment table, DMAIC projects logically strung together can have an unparalleled impact on strategic results for quality, throughput, patient safety, and cost recovery.

Although the Cost of Quality recovery potential will be driven by the size of the organization, a midsized organization should establish thresholds close to suggestions in Table 3.1.

Table 3.1   Comparison of DMAIC, PDCA, and 100-Day Workout.

Method	Duration	Process improvement potential	Minimum cost of quality recovery
DMAIC	4–6 months	10-fold	> $150,000
PDCA	12 weeks	15% to 25%	> $100,000
100-Day Workout	100 days	5% to 15%	> $ 75,000
Manager project	Varies	< 5%	Varies

DMAIC

Define-measure-analyze-improve-control (DMAIC) is the main workhorse of the four Lean-Six Sigma methods and can be thought of as "PDCA on steroids." Typically, DMAIC is the appropriate method when you believe there is the potential for a 10-fold process improvement with at least $300,000 annualized cost recovery potential the first year and $150,000 in later years.

Although the underlying quality improvement logic of DMAIC is similar to basic performance improvement methods, a significant number of additional tools are used with DMAIC. In addition to the basics, DMAIC's prowess encompasses the following characteristics above and beyond performance improvement methods such as PDCA.

Advanced Customer Knowledge Discovery

Unlike traditional improvement methodologies, which focus mainly on averages and medians, DMAIC requires more intimate knowledge of customer needs, as discussed in Chapter 2. Specifically, we need to determine the performance limit beyond which unacceptable quality levels repel customers. In other words, at what point do our customers feel our organization has begun providing poor quality?

In DMAIC language, this limit is revealed through the upper specification limit, or USL. The USL is the point beyond which customers will be disgusted with your performance. The USL can perhaps best be thought of as a measured "Voice of the Customer" (Pande 2000, 176–184). For example, patients may expect to be treated in the emergency department within 120 minutes, but they will walk out after 150 minutes. Or, the acceptable quality for acute myocardial infarction (MI) patients might be to receive a beta blocker within 12 hours of presentation, and poor quality is defined as greater than 24 hours. Of course, if the "direction" of quality is upward instead of downward (for example, you use the percentage of acute MI patients receiving a beta blocker within 24 hours), the key measure is reversed and labeled the lower specification limit, or LSL.

To grasp the full view of customer expectations and relate the importance of selected processes and features in terms of Cost of Quality, Rust (1994) advocates the widespread use of customer focus groups, both internal and external. The use of focus groups need not be sophisticated endeavors, as used by marketing professionals, but rather informal discussions about the characteristics and flow of the desired future state compared to the current state.

Predictive Statistics to Determine Key Process Drivers

Once we have determined the USL (and/or LSL, as appropriate) and gained process capability knowledge, DMAIC provides a set of tools to determine subprocess importance to the USL. These tools, such as regression analysis and analysis of variation (ANOVA), are typically used by leading patient satisfaction firms when they provide a list of those factors that, if improved, would more likely improve overall satisfaction than if other factors were improved. DMAIC brings that level of sophistication to all our process improvement efforts.

Use of the Lean-Six Sigma Solution Set

Concepts for design change are used in some DMAIC versions to stimulate creativity beyond simple benchmarking. Popularized by leading thinker Tom Nolan and his colleagues, "change concepts," as he refers to them, are generalized notions of design that have the effect of reducing waste, improving throughput and cycle times, and recovering costs (Langley 1996). These design solutions enable executives and others to coach in the actual design concepts that can be applied to improve processes. Refer to Chapter 2 for a listing of the broad Lean-Six Sigma solution set outlining change concepts and to Appendix C for a complete digest of more than 50 solutions; additionally, an electronic version is on the CD and available for download from www.chipcaldwellassoc.com/resources. Other techniques for creativity include mind mapping, a process of linking ideas, and synectics, a process of building a solution from an unrelated innovation (Weintraub 1998).

Rapid Cycle Experiments to Validate the Effectiveness of Process Changes

 Experimentation tools such as design of experiments (DOE) (Pyzdek 2001) are used in DMAIC to help determine whether theories about interventions to improve process performance are accurate. Most healthcare executives are familiar with the logic of PDCA, or plan-do-check-act, although rarely do PDCA projects, even those using FOCUS-PDCA, effectively use a PDCA testing cycle. Performance improvement models validate these process intervention tests, but DMAIC takes experimentation a step further by using DOE tools, and it contains significant rigor in the testing phase. Certain DOE tools, such as two-sample t-tests and factorial analysis, allow leaders to test several theories simultaneously, saving both time and money. Regardless of the tool deployed, the DMAIC distinction is rigorous tests of change effectiveness against the original hypotheses. As pointed out by Tom Nolan (Langley 1996), tests of change are most effective if conducted quickly after the change—one shift, one day, three days, one week. Rarely is it necessary to test longer than one week unless the process is performed only infrequently.

An example of a rapid cycle experiment in an ED might be the desire to test the effectiveness of advance protocols implemented by triage nurses versus waiting until the patient is assessed by the ED physician later in the care process. To test this change, a Black Belt will set up the experiment by conducting a baseline, followed by a very rapid test of the change to be tested, in this case, advance protocols. Figure 3.1 provides the results of the test over a three-day period.

As Figure 3.1 demonstrates, the presence of advance protocols makes an obvious difference in "time to orders."

A tenet of rapid cycle experimentation is to conduct the test of change as quickly as possible. Traditional statistical sampling theory suggests that very large sample sizes are required to determine the effectiveness of a

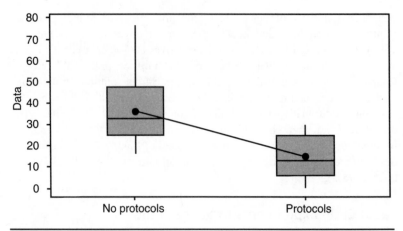

Figure 3.1   Boxplot of advance protocols on triage-to-orders time.

change, but the initial test need not be delayed until a large sample size is amassed. Tom Nolan suggests that rapid experiments over the next shift, the next day, or the next three days using 25 data points is desirable over tests requiring three months and more than 400 data points and that such large sample sizes, while perhaps in conformance to the rigor of statistical theory, necessitate delays in rapidly executing and moving to the next test of change (Langley 1996). As Figure 3.1 illustrates, testing the effectiveness of advance protocols over one shift demonstrates that they are effective under the circumstances present during that shift. The main issue remaining, then, is to what degree that shift represents ED patient care under all circumstances. If representativeness is at issue, subsequent tests can be conducted if the first experiment passes.

Managers at all levels can benefit from being trained in rapid cycle experiments to ensure that a process change has resulted in an improvement and that any additional resources added to the process, even outside of DMAIC. This skill set would prevent many process changes that require additional costs, such as added FTEs, when the return on these additional costs is minimal. Rapid cycle experimentation skills need not be restricted to Black Belts.

While the triage example illustrates a single change tested independently, as recommended by Nolan as long as the experiment is conducted rapidly, such as over the next shift, the noted statistician George Box (1978) points out that simultaneous testing of several potential changes is more efficient than testing each potential change one at a time. Therefore, at some point, factorial analysis and Lean-Six Sigma simulation techniques must be brought into the DMAIC tool kit.

Error-Proofing Pilots of Change

Tools such as failure modes effects analysis (FMEA), a longtime technique used by engineers and Black Belts and popularized for patient care staff by the Joint Commission on Accreditation of Healthcare Organizations (JCAHO), and poka yoke, a Japanese term for mistake-proofing, are used for error detection and error proofing and error mitigation (Pande 2000, 372–375). As change pilots are concluded, DMAIC expects that events highly probable of producing a variation in quality will be uncovered. These events are called failure modes. Dr. Joseph Juran's Quality Control Spreadsheet is another tool (Juran 1994). As failures are predicted, the organization is expected to deploy tools and processes both to detect that an error is eminent and to prevent it. Or if the error has already occurred, it should be detected quickly and its adverse effects mitigated before the error becomes catastrophic or costly.

A manufacturing example involves a component that requires four rivets. Rather than relying on the memory of a technician to always install the correct number, four rivets would be placed in a small plastic bowl before installation. Upon completion of the riveting, if any rivets remain in the bowl, then obviously an error occurred. Similar processes exist in surgery to ensure that surgical sponges are removed before the incision is closed. Another example is the use of audible alarms on IV infusion systems.

Use of MINITAB® Statistical Software

Although one could manipulate the formulas and data sets used in DMAIC manually, who would want to? Some of us still remember the slide rule. Several popular software packages are available, the most popular being MINITAB®, which can dramatically expedite the analysis process.

The general steps found in most DMAIC models appear in Figure 3.2.

PDCA-TYPE METHOD

While the DMAIC method is most appropriate when initial analysis suggests a strong probability for a 10-fold subprocess yield improvement and a $150,000 to $500,000 cost recovery potential, the PDCA (plan-do-check-act) method would be the best choice if you anticipate only a 25% process improvement with $100,000 to $150,000 cost recovery.

Many healthcare leaders may know about certain PDCA-type methods, such as Paul Batalden's FOCUS-PDCA (Caldwell 2004a) or Tom Nolan's Aim-Measure PDSA (plan-do-study-act) (Langley 1996), but most senior

Phase	Step	Description	Questions answered
		Formulate/Describe the Practical Opportunity	
Define	A	Identify project CTQ's	What's important to my customer?
	B	Develop team charter	What am I going to do about it? How?
	C	Define Process Map	What is my area of focus?
Measure	1	Select CTQ characteristics	What issues can I measure/improve?
	2	Define performance standards	What does "good" performance look like?
	3	Validate measurement system	Are my measurement reliable/useful?
		Convert the Opportunity to a Statistical Problem	
Analyze	4	Eastable process capabilities	How good am I today?
	5	Define performance objectives	How good do I need to be?
	6	Identify variation sources	What factors affect performance?
		Solve the Statistical Problem	
Improve	7	Screen potential causes	Which factors can I leverage to improve?
	8	Discover variable reslationships	How can I predict outcomes?
	9	Establish operating tolerances	How tight/consistent must control be?
		Implement the Practical Solution	
Control	10	Define and validate measurement of X's	Can I get an accurate read on key factors?
	11	Determine process capability	Have I reached my goal?
	12	Implement process control	What must be done to sustain improvements?

Figure 3.2 DMAIC steps.

Source: Dunn, Terry, General Electric, and Chip Caldwell. 2004. "Six Sigma for Healthcare Organizations." Paper presented at the National Managed Care Congress, Washington, May 5, 2004. Used with permission.

executives and many managers have abandoned the logic of their initial quality management efforts. This industrywide abandonment is certainly understandable, considering the early burdensome approach to PDCA deployment when the effort was more to ensure that everyone had a flow-chart, a cause-and-effect diagram, and a Pareto chart than to achieve a critical result.

In the end, managers resisted this approach to management problem solving because too often each tool was not necessary for achieving the strategic result. This approach was somewhat like a carpenter insisting that his apprentices use every tool in their belts, even if the tool was not needed.

Regardless, the logic of PDCA as a problem-solving approach for managers has not been bested in more than 70 years. As Juran (1994) observed, it is a diagnostic-remedial process so familiar to clinicians that is applied to management thinking. Or as some have stated, it is "management by fact."

Several key disciplines must be present in any PDCA method for the effort exerted to match the strategic potential. They are:

- *Strategically aligned mission or charter*—Is the mission clear? Is it obvious which strategic priority aligns with it? Will the results be measurable? Have we expressed the time frame within which the result is expected? Is the goal a stretch goal, or is it a comfortable one? Have senior leaders cleared the way for allied process owners to support the effort, or will the team be likely frustrated by resistance?

- *Process knowledge discovery*—Does our PDCA approach ensure that the manager and/or team understand the underlying subprocesses and their metrics, or are we assuming again?

- *Process variation root cause analysis*—Does our approach provide a rich set of data to ensure that the team aims at the high leverage subprocesses and performance drivers? Or are we at risk that they might work on the "small stuff"?

- *Creative process integration*—Does our method ensure that the managers and/or teams first develop a potential process intervention criteria matrix, and second, brainstorm at least five potential interventions? Or does our method permit preconceived solutions?

- *Active experimentation*—Does our approach provide for a time-limited pilot, after which performance metrics are assessed against the original project mission? Or does it permit process tampering and then acting as though the project is complete without assessment?

- *Hold the gains*—Does our process contain a way for successful pilots to become part of day-to-day work, such as a form to include the date that policy manuals were changed, training was conducted, and/or department-level quality control spreadsheets or failure modes effects analysis spreadsheets were deployed?

- *PDCA improvement*—Does our process contain a request that the manager assess the PDCA effort just completed and make recommendations to improve the use of PDCA throughout the organization?

- *Speed*—Did the manager complete the project within 90 days?

A template to assess effectiveness of an organization's use of PDCA-type methods is available in Appendix D and on the CD.

100-DAY WORKOUT METHOD

The 100-Day Workout is an execution-oriented methodology (Caldwell 2004a). Traditional improvement models devote the least amount of time to implementation, whereas effective models devote at least 25% of time to implementation (Mozena 1999). The 100-Day Workout allocates over 75% to implementation. General Electric, which popularized the Workout methodology, even uses the methodology with suppliers and customers (Senge 1999, 77). Compared to other methods, effective deployment of 100-Day Workout will require the greatest transformation among managers about the best way to manage the organization. 100-Day Workout is the best Lean-Six Sigma improvement methodology to choose when your organization already possesses a workable solution set and anticipates a 5% to 15% process improvement with a $75,000 cost recovery.

Typically, as organizational strategy deployment discussions lead to project selection and formation, managers who are selected to execute the various projects deploy a protracted process that can take as long as six months and almost never is completed within 90 days. This project deployment process involves assembling key managers and staff critical to the project's success, articulating various execution strategies, assigning homework to be completed before the next meeting, and meeting again in two to four weeks. At the follow-up meeting, managers present their initial thinking, sometimes labeled "draft," receive input from their colleagues, and then take another 30 days to get organized. Rarely does the organization possess a standardized, disciplined process, structure, or reporting format for the projects, but rather it leaves structural considerations up to the individual manager or vice president. Managers usually begin to calendar the steps necessary to actually execute process changes. Time constraints, resistance, other emerging priorities, and the lessening sense of urgency that occurs as time passes usually result in another 30 to 60 days before any meaningful process intervention is made.

The 100-Day Workout turns this world upside down. It is an invigorating, execution-driven process in which process interventions begin immediately, not after any protracted period. The 100-Day Workout session template is scheduled to last 2½ to 3½ days, but it can be stretched into four meetings over two weeks if required. In some cases, the kickoff can be conducted in one day, but be cautious with reducing the session to a planning-only session. A foundational aspect of a 100-Day Workout is execution, execution, execution. Any period greater than two weeks between action planning and the completion of the first implemented change reclassifies the 100-Day Workout to a manager project, having lost the 100-Day Workout's critical characteristics of speed and execution.

The original 100-Day Workout template, created by Sherry Bright for Chip Caldwell and Associates, follows several steps.

100-Day Workout Goal Clarification— Two to Four Weeks before Kickoff

Senior executives charter the 100-Day Workout based on clearly defined and measured strategic priorities. A critical success factor is clarity of objectives; unclear objectives or objectives that lack senior management's resolve to achieve will scuttle the 100-Day Workout experience. Next, senior executives appoint an accountable senior leader champion, a 100-Day Workout manager (usually a department manager), and a 100-Day Workout facilitator.

Pre-work—About 14 Days' Duration, One to Four Weeks before Kickoff

For the 100-Day Workout session to be successful, planning is vital. First, a 100-Day Workout week is calendared, and all attendees block off this time in their calendars. There can be no exceptions. The senior executive sponsor must clear the way for other priorities to be managed by someone else and/or delayed until the 100-Day Workout is complete. The 100-Day Workout facilitator, with assistance from the 100-Day Workout manager, helps establish expectations for all participants, including calendaring meetings in advance. The 100-Day Workout manager and others complete a high-level flowchart of the process under discussion and assemble all available data about performance of the process. Known gaps in data are filled, using sampling techniques. Of particular concern are data revealing quality yield, sigma levels, total cost, and Cost of Quality.

Yield refers to the percentage conformance to quality. For example, the national average for beta blocker administration within 24 hours for acute MI patients rests at 61% (Caldwell 2001). This yield equals a sigma value of 1.8 Sigma. The yield for x-ray exams is about 93% (or its invert, 7% retakes), or Three Sigma. The yield for medication administration is about 90%, according to Lucian Leape's report (Caldwell 2001), which equates to 2.8 Sigma. Cost of Quality, as noted previously, is the cost, particularly FTEs, that is invested to inspect for presence of these "misses" and that is involved in the rework to reverse the negative effects of the errors. In most processes, approximately 14% of the total cost is tied up in inspection-based work and 20% can be attributed to rework.

The last pre-work task for the 100-Day Workout manager and facilitator is to assemble a Lean-Six Sigma solution set database from literature review and benchmarking calls. A defined structure for the Lean-Six Sigma solution set database has been defined by international quality leader Tom Nolan (Langley 1996, 294).

100-Day Workout Kickoff—2½–3½ Days

- *Monday.* The session typically begins on a Monday morning. From initiation until noon, the 100-Day Workout manager and facilitator review and seek consensus on the precise objectives of the 100-Day Workout, the high-level flowchart, and current performance measures, and then they determine any data gaps that might exist. 100-Day Workout participants adjourn for the remainder of the day to collect data samples to close identified gaps, using predesigned forms.

- *Tuesday.* The 100-Day Workout reconvenes on Tuesday morning with brief presentations of data collected Monday afternoon. The 100-Day Workout manager then leads a root cause analysis discussion. If the process contains more than three subprocesses, participants can be broken up into work teams. During this three-hour assessment, some participants might leave the 100-Day Workout to gather data or past reports and bring them back into the 100-Day Workout. Whether or not the root cause analysis is complete at noon, the 100-Day Workout progresses to the solution phase. The 100-Day Workout manager presents the solution set created in the pre-work, and participants commit to specific process interventions. It is important that interventions be broken into bite-size process changes, not "solve world hunger" changes. With one hour remaining in the day, participants divide interventions into three categories, as follows:

– *Do Now*. These are process interventions that will be completed before the week's end. As the Do Now designation is applied, participants agree on who will take charge of implementation during the next few hours. This is a very important distinction of 100-Day Workout. It actually means "complete implementation now," not "begin to implement now."

– *Complete in 30 days*. These are the process changes that will be initiated within the next few days, but they will be completed by the first 30-day check-in meeting.

– *Complete in 60 days*. These are the process changes that will be initiated within the next few days, but they will be completed within 60 days.

– *Complete in 90 days*. These are the process changes that will be initiated within the next few days, but they will be completed within 90 days.

– Ideas consuming greater than 90 days, while not necessarily unimportant, are removed from the agenda because the 100-Day Workout aims for 90-day completion.

• *Wednesday–Thursday noon*. The 100-Day Workout is adjourned while participants complete the Do Now list and initiate the longer-term interventions.

• *Thursday afternoon*. The 100-Day Workout reconvenes with reports by participants regarding their executions. Unknowable factors might necessitate moving a Do Now intervention into the 30-day category, but these reclassifications must be exceedingly rare.

In some instances, the kickoff can be abbreviated to a one-day session, with a "Do Now" check-in conducted within two to three days to ensure rapid implementation.

30-Day Check-Ins

Three check-in sessions of three hours each occur at 30-day intervals to ensure progress is being made and barriers are being removed.

Day 1	• Introduction • Waste and waste elimination tools • 2-hour "Waste Walk" • Construct Do Nows, 30-, 60-, 90-day change lists, and execution plan
Day 2	• Execute Do Nows

Day 3	• Execution (continued)
	• Present Do Nows completed and 30-, 60-, and 90-day plans to CEO/COO
	• Next meeting dates/steps
	    ✍ 30-day check-in
	    ✍ 60-day check-in
	    ✍ 90-day check-in
	    ✍ Summation/Kick off next 100-Day Workout

Figure 3.3   100-Day Workout agenda.

Summation

The final three-hour meeting, occurring about 120 days (allowing 100 days to implement and 20 days to analyze bottom-line results) after the 100-Day Workout begins, concludes the 100-Day Workout. The 100-Day Workout manager and facilitator present updated performance data on yield, sigma levels, projected total cost, and Cost of Quality recovery, including FTEs reassigned or reduced.

Figure 3.3 illustrates a specific type of 100-Day Workout known as an Operations Waste 100-Day Workout. This aggressive cost recovery project method has produced over $1 million (annualized) in most organizations (Caldwell 2004a).

MANAGER PROJECT

The manager project is actually a catchall category for projects that do not fit the project selection matrix criteria for the DMAIC, PDCA, or 100-Day Workout. However, Lean-Six Sigma organizations strengthen their manager project methods by adding a standardized, disciplined project management process and format. Disciplined adherence to the use of Microsoft Project, or similar project management software, along with project management training and coaching can only accelerate the magnitude of improvements made by managers.

ASSESSING CURRENT IMPROVEMENT METHODS

Every organization should assess its project methods annually, looking to upgrade and improve the effectiveness of the ways improvements are discovered, implemented, and hardwired. This is especially true for an organization that is new to Lean-Six Sigma or that has initiated a Lean-Six Sigma initiative in the past couple of years. An assessment tool can be found in Appendix D, or in electronic version on the CD or website, to help determine an organization's current state.

No two organizations are identical. Some organizations possess strengths of strategic alignment; others possess strengths of project launching, while others excel at execution. To determine which methods should be contained in your Lean-Six Sigma suite, begin with an honest self-assessment of the strengths and weaknesses of the improvement methods your organization uses every day.

The adage "Don't throw the baby out with the bath water" could not be more appropriate when considering how to evolve an organization's existing approach to achieving strategic results to Lean-Six Sigma performance. Every sound improvement method, whether off-the-shelf like PDCA or your own homegrown method, contains basic characteristics, which can be discovered through manager interviews and background data assimilation.

When accessing the strengths and weaknesses of an organization's existing improvement methods, look for these basics:

- Strategically aligned project charter. Improvement projects always must be aligned with strategic goals, rather than being unrelated, nonstrategic efforts haphazardly initiated. A project charter that follows a SMART mission statement framework is an excellent way to make that happen:

  - Specifically boundaried process

  - Measured results

  - Agreed upon by the project team, the senior management champion, and the executive steering committee if one exists

  - Realistic, yet stretch improvement expected

  - Time-based

  For example, a SMART mission statement for a Lean-Six Sigma project might be "To achieve a 10-fold improvement in critical care unit adverse drug events, from 1.8% discharges to 0.18%, by April 1," or "To achieve a 10-fold improvement,

from 7% yield (Zero Sigma) to 70% (Two Sigma) in the
revenue cycle auto-adjudication process in six months."

- A process discovery technique. Successful improvement
methods include a process discovery technique that generates a
comprehensive understanding of process boundaries, profound
knowledge of customers served by the process, and current
performance against customer expectations compared to the
SMART mission of the project team. Most often this
characteristic is accomplished by using a flowchart, but one of
the failings of the early quality improvement movement was to
focus on presence of specific tools rather than the underlying
discipline. Actually, how process knowledge is gained is more
important than mandating the use of a specific tool.

- Process variation root cause analysis. The most common tools
used to understand the root cause of process variation are
cause-and-effect analysis followed by a Pareto chart. Again,
it is more important to probe openly for how root causes are
uncovered than to use specific charts and graphs. Managers
creatively adapt tools to their unique staff cultures without
necessarily destroying the validity of preferred tool sets.

- Creative process intervention. Once process performance
variation drivers have been determined, an effective
improvement method leads the project team to develop a listing
of potential interventions to eliminate the greatest causes of
variation or to mitigate the harmful effects of the variation. Of
all the assessments we have conducted over the years, root
cause analysis and potential interventions are the most common
to be cut short. Teams prefer, it seems, to immediately launch a
predetermined "best idea" without taking full advantage of the
creative process. The most common tool for this purpose, of
course, is brainstorming. Once the potential interventions list
is created, an effective improvement method leads the team to
establish intervention selection prioritization criteria so that
pilots can be initiated.

- Active experiment validation method. As best-guess
interventions are determined, a process to test the intervention
under field, or real world, conditions is necessary to validate
underlying assumptions about the intervention's effectiveness.
Most often, this step involves the use of a plan-do-check-act
cycle. Absence of this intervention validation cycle is the
second most commonly omitted feature we have found during
our assessments.

- Hold the gains/hardwiring solutions. Once a process intervention has proven effective, it is time to turn over the ongoing assessment of the new level of performance to operating units. This is usually accomplished via the department's monthly quality control activities, but, in the absence of effective department-level quality control, it can be stimulated through the annual strategic planning process.

- Improvement project cycle time. The assessment should test for the average cycle time between and during performance improvement projects. An effective departmental method that requires an average of six months to complete, followed by a 90-day break, produces radically different results over three years than a department with a model capable of sustaining a change every 90 days, with only a few days' lag time between.

An example of a completed performance improvement assessment is shown in Figure 3.4.

The importance of conducting such a self-assessment before launching a Lean-Six Sigma initiative or within the first two years of execution cannot be overemphasized. Successful evolution to the more rigorous methods required of Lean-Six Sigma depends upon a stable foundation of these basics before more advanced tools can be added to the organization's tool kit. After conducting a baseline assessment and creating a roadmap, tasks are generally divided into two categories:

- *Sharpen the saw*—These tasks close gaps among the basics and ensure stabilization so that quantum improvement can be realized as Lean-Six Sigma tools are added.

- *Quantum improvement*—These tasks advance the organization to the next level of Lean-Six Sigma.

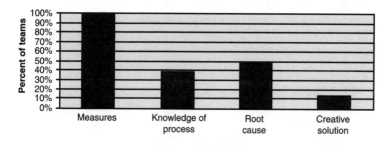

Figure 3.4   Quality system assessment.

Once senior leaders determine that improvement efforts are strategically aligned and existing improvement methods are fully assessed, they are ready to add more advanced methods to their tool bag.

SUMMARY

Lean-Six Sigma's four project methods, particularly DMAIC and the 100-Day Workout, exert a powerful array of opportunity identification, discipline, and measurable bottom-line results. However, it is a critical role of senior leadership not to become statisticians or engineers, but to own and ensure effective deployment of these powerful methods within the organization's strategic framework, as will be reviewed in detail in Chapter 4.

CHECKLISTS AND TOOLS ACCESSIBLE ELECTRONICALLY

- Lean-Six Sigma Solution Set—see Appendix C and the CD.
- PDCA Project Method Assessment template—Appendix D or access the CD.
- 100-Day Workout template—access the CD.

RECOMMENDED LEARNING SESSIONS

Learning Session for a One-Hour Senior Leader Meeting

Pre-work. Three weeks before the senior leader team meeting, commission a quality professional, management engineer, or analyst, in concert with an executive team member, to conduct an assessment of the last 10 completed projects; include both operations projects and DRG (Diagnostic Related Groups) based projects. Using the PDCA Project Method Assessment Workpaper found in Appendix D, this assessment should be made available to the executive team one week before the session.

In addition, acquire a run chart of monthly performance over the past 24 months in the following areas:

- Top 12 DRGs by volume—run chart cost per discharge.
  Use charges if cost accounted data is unavailable; charges will
  be relevant for this analysis because we are benchmarking
  ourselves over time.
- Worked hours per unit of service.

The One-hour Senior Leader Meeting. One member of the executive team should serve as the recorder, capturing feedback on a flipchart. The quality professional, management engineer, or analyst and the executive partner should present a high-level overview of the run charts and the projects reviewed. During the next hour, address the following questions:

1. Has our performance improved according to the run charts? Do we wish for them to improve?

2. What strengths exist in our current project methods? How can these strengths be replicated in parts of the organization that are not optimizing them?

3. What are our weaknesses? How can we reduce these weaknesses?

REFERENCES

Box, George, William Hunter, and Stuart Hunter. 1978. *Statistics for Experimenters.* New York: John Wiley & Sons, 4.

Breyfogle, Forrest. 2003. *Implementing Six Sigma,* 2nd edition. Hoboken, NJ: John Wiley & Sons.

Caldwell, Chip. 2004. "Good to Great in Healthcare: A Research Initiative." Conference presented by the American College of Healthcare Executives, St. Louis, May 26, 2004.

Caldwell, Chip, and James Brexler. 2004. "Improving Throughput and Costs Using Lean-Six Sigma." Conference presented by the American College of Healthcare Executives, Key West, FL, January 12–13, 2004.

Caldwell, Chip, and Charles Denham. 2001. *Medication Safety and Cost Recovery: A Four-Step Approach for Executives.* Chicago: Health Administration Press.

Caldwell, Chip, and Bruce Tilley. 2004. "Aggressive Cost Reduction Using Lean-Six Sigma." National teleconference presented by the VHA and the American College of Healthcare Executives, Dallas, March 25, 2004.

Dunn, Terry, and Chip Caldwell. 2004. "Six Sigma for Healthcare Organizations." Paper presented at the National Managed Care Congress, Washington, May 5, 2004.

Healthcare Advisory Board. 1999. *The Clockwork ED.* Washington: Advisory Board Company.

Juran, Joseph. 1994. "Develop Process Controls—Transfer to Operations". *Designs for Worldclass Quality.* Wilton, CT: Juran Institute.

Langley, Gerald, Kevin Nolan, Thomas Nolan, Clifford Norman, and Lloyd Provost. 1996. *The Improvement Guide.* San Francisco: Jossey-Bass Publishers.

Mozena, James, Charles Emerick, and Steve Black. 1999. *Stop Managing Costs.* Milwaukee: ASQ Quality Press, 37–38.

Pande, Peter, Robert Neuman, and Roland Cavanagh. 2000. *The Six Sigma Way.* New York: McGraw Hill.

Pyzdek, Thomas. 2001. *The Six Sigma Handbook*. New York: McGraw Hill.

Rust, Roland, Anthony Zahorik, and Timothy Keiningham. 1994. *Return on Quality*. Chicago: Probus Publishing.

Senge, Peter, Art Kleiner, Charlotte Roberts, Richard Ross, George Roth, and Bryan Smith. 1999. *The Dance of Change*. New York: Currency Doubleday.

Weintraub, Sandra. 1998. *The Hidden Intelligence*. Boston: Butterworth Heinemann.

ADDITIONAL READING

Pande, Peter, Robert Neuman, and Roland Cavanagh. 2000. *The Six Sigma Way*. New York: McGraw Hill.

Pyzdek, Thomas. 2001. *The Six Sigma Handbook*. New York: McGraw Hill.

4

The Role of Senior Leaders: Achieving the Strategic Magic Moment

If at first you don't succeed,
find out if the loser gets anything.

Bill Lyon

The leader's role is to manage the Magic Moment. This declaration made sense to the senior executives who heard Heartland Health chief operating officer Curt Kretzinger coin the term, and it resonates clearly with most other executive teams as well. It is not the role of senior leaders to come together to charter Lean-Six Sigma teams and listen to their detailed project reports. Rather, it is the role of senior leaders to build and maintain the infrastructure in which strategic results come together at some future point.

The role of senior leaders is often misunderstood or misapplied in Lean-Six Sigma launches. Many of the leading texts on the subject do little to steer leaders in the right direction. For example, some texts say the role of leaders is to determine the criteria for Black Belt nomination and select and oversee their progress. Others suggest that leaders be involved in the detailed review of the specific path within a DMAIC project, including review of statistical analyses and root cause analysis.

While there is nothing inherently incorrect about leaders learning from this low level of engagement, it is the primary reason, however, that senior leaders disengage from the implementation of Lean-Six Sigma after only a few short months. Project review is not the work of senior leaders, and they quickly tire or become immersed in more strategic issues and begin to miss meetings. Barry (2004), a leading healthcare Lean-Six Sigma thinker, amplifies this point. "The many-versus-few choice is up to the organization's senior management. We personally recommend fewer projects." So if Black Belt selection and project review is not the domain of leaders, what is?

The short answer is one role of senior leaders, as reviewed in Chapter 1, is to ensure that Lean-Six Sigma is deployed as a powerful strategic results engine—to ensure that the Magic Moment happens. To manage the Magic Moment, leaders must engage in seven distinct leadership activities:

1. Clearly articulate the strategic aims of the Lean-Six Sigma effort as it relates to the long-term vision and three- to five-year goals, at the integrated delivery network (IDN) level, organization level, and core process level.

2. Translate core process cost recovery goals into process goals as a basis for Lean-Six Sigma project determination.

3. Create and maintain an organization system map highlighting the interrelationships between core functional processes within the organization and their specific three- to five-year goals aimed at achieving the organization's overall three- to five-year goals.

4. Assign key accountable executives to each core functional process who create and implement internal metrics; charter Lean-Six Sigma project teams; appoint project leaders and Black Belts to ensure rapid implementation of identified, high-leverage process improvements; and adjust plans according to progress toward the three- to five-year goals.

5. Deploy a Lean-Six Sigma Resource Group to manage the necessary infrastructure and project schedule to carry out those aims.

6. Measure progress toward three- to five-year strategic results using advanced techniques such as the balanced scorecard or other measurement template.

7. Aggressively track project milestones that have been commissioned by executive leaders.

These tasks must be exceptionally well managed, and they are nondelegable. That is, no one can substitute for the role of senior leaders in the organization for achieving quantum results and managing the Magic Moment.

ACHIEVING THE MAGIC MOMENT

Setting Lean-Six Sigma Cost Goals

As with any significant strategic effort, the "ends" must be clearly articulated, measured, and communicated before the "means" can be determined.

A key characteristic of a Lean-Six Sigma deployment is that leaders establish the roadmap for strategic results and manage the infrastructure required to get there. It is not a role of the senior leadership team to charter projects or even to follow progress of chartered teams. The task of project determination and project tracking, as will be discussed in the Senior Leader Missteps section later in this chapter, is best left to individual VPs who are accountable to achieve a specific strategy. Stated another way, accountability should acknowledge what we accomplish, not how busy we are.

The most critical question is, "What do we wish to achieve over the next three to five years?" And, yet, this question is often not asked at the time of project selection; instead the question often is, "What project ideas do we have and what is the best one to initiate now?"

The layout of the Magic Moment spreadsheet, shown in Figure 4.1 (and available on CD and for download according to the instructions found at the end of the chapter), provides a vital planning visual for the executive team.

Magic Moment planning begins with the determination of those core processes that make up the organization and are large enough to warrant significant project activity and assignment to an accountable executive. Typical selections by executive teams, designated "1" in the first column of the Magic Moment spreadsheet template in Figure 4.1, are operations (representing the functional departments of the organization), patient care throughput, surgery, care optimization/clinical decision making, revenue cycle, ED, registration, diagnostic services, and therapeutic services. Assigned to each core process are an accountable executive, usually designated by an officer or vice president title, and a 0.5 full-time equivalent Black Belt, a role to be defined later in the chapter.

Secondly, the planning horizon for each wave of projects is 100 days to six months, designated "2" in Figure 4.1.

Each of these DMAIC and 100-Day Workout projects is budgeted to recover a minimum amount of Cost of Quality, totaling a specific threshold during each wave, shown as "3" in Figure 4.1. Projects sometimes exceed the project thresholds and sometimes they fall short.

Finally, the Magic Moment results, shown as "4" in Figure 4.1, enable executive leaders to determine whether the overall strategic goal is being met.

While the structure forecasts and tracks Cost of Quality recovery as a result of waste removal and throughput improvement, the same structure can be used for improvements in patient satisfaction and other nonfinancial goals, although with slightly more difficulty.

Key Process	1st-Half FY ②	SAVINGS	ACT	2nd-Half FT	SAVINGS	ACT	PLANNED ACT	ACTUAL Cums To Date
Operations ① (VP and Black Belt)	DMAIC	0.300	0.295	DMAIC	0.300	0.350		
	100-Day WO	0.075	1.025	100-Day WO	0.075	0.875	0.750	2.545
Patient Care (VP and Black Belt)	DMAIC	0.300	0.325	DMAIC	0.300	0.106		
	100-Day WO	0.075	0.080	100-Day WO	0.075	0.125	0.750	0.636
Surgery (VP and Black Belt)	DMAIC	0.300	0.495	DMAIC	0.300	0.451		
	100-Day WO	0.075	0.100	100-Day WO	0.075	0.050	0.750	1.096
Care Optimization (VP and Black Belt)	DMAIC	0.300	1.800	DMAIC	0.300	0.675		
	100-Day WO	0.075	0.050	100-Day WO	0.075	0.140	0.750	2.665
Rev Cycle (VP and Black Belt)	DMAIC	0.300	0.410	DMAIC	0.300	1.100		
	100-Day WO	0.075	0.210	100-Day WO	0.075	0.030	0.750	1.750
SAVINGS TOTALS		$ 1.4 ③	$ 4.8		$ 1.4	$ 3.9	3.750	④ $ 8.7
SAVINGS TOTALS * 75%		$ 1.4	$ 4.8		2.8	$ 8.7	2.8	$ 8.7
CUM TOTALS								

Figure 4.1   Magic Moment strategy deployment spreadsheet.

Translate Core Care and Business Cost Goals into Process Goals

Conveying core process Cost of Quality recovery goals alone to accountable senior leaders, department directors, and clinical leaders without also providing an agreed-upon process-specific framework within which these leaders will operate has proven to be an ineffective route to achieve sustainable cost advantage. Simply alerting a department director that she was seven full-time equivalent staff higher than the benchmark ceased to provide the level of support required in the current operating environment to extract costs that are sustainable. The lack of additional support for leaders to translate cost goals into process goals has led to frustration and suboptimal results over the last couple of years. Lean-Six Sigma concepts are ideally suited to aid executives and department directors in determining those high-leverage process focus areas, that, if improved, will yield cost recovery as the exhaust of their efforts, as discussed in Chapter 2. The suggested senior leader and manager learning sessions at the end of this chapter can be helpful in translating these concepts into actions. While many cost goals can easily be converted into their process waste and throughput drivers, many functional areas are more elusive. Table 4.1 provides a starting point for accountable executives to begin the process of translating their assigned core process goals into process goals.

The importance of the establishment and continual evolution of the translation process cannot be overstated and, like many other components of the Magic Moment, is a nondelegable task of senior leaders.

Core Care and Business Process Mapping

To ensure there is a strategic line of sight, a care/business process map, often called a system map, must be linked to strategic goals. Clearly aligned strategic goals expected from the Lean-Six Sigma effort in measurable terms to the three- to five-year goals contained in the organization's strategic plan is foundational in the sense that if we fail to articulate and measure our goals effectively, everything that follows contains no strategic meaning. Most healthcare strategic plans are quite specific regarding three- to five-year expectations for patient satisfaction results, patient safety results, and financial performance. These strategic focus areas are ideally suited for Lean-Six Sigma application. It is becoming more common to see patient care throughput, ED throughput, and surgery throughput goals contained within organizations' strategic plans and these goals are strongly correlated with Lean-Six Sigma strengths.

Through care and business process mapping, the organization leaders can discover and communicate the interrelationships, at the organizational

Table 4.1   Core care and business process translation workplan. (An electronic version can be found on the CD.)

Core Process	Cost Recovery Goal	Process Translation Goal	Observable Impact
Operations Waste Management	Top quartile cost per department unit of service (e.g. 3.5 FTEs per Adjusted Occupied Bed)	• Close 20% staffing-demand curve gap • Waste Walk—10 improvements per 100 days	• Fewer worked hours per week in each department • Fewer worked hours per department unit of service
ED	Top quartile cost per ED visit (e.g. 1.8 worked hours per ED visit versus current 2.8)	• LOS to USL of 4 hours (versus current 6 hours) (saving 0.5 worked hours per ED visit) • Left without treatment (LWOT) to 0.5% from 2.5% • Diversions to less then 1 hour per week from current 1 hour per day • ED Admitted Patients Request For Bed within 30-min of ED physician initial assessment.	• Fewer worked hour per week, particularly RN hours • Lower LWOTs and diversion hours
Surgery	Top quartile cost per surgery case	• "Cut-close" hours / staffed hours to 85% (from 70% current) • 1st case start time at 4-Sigma (from 2-Sigma) • To-follow at 4-Sigma (from 1.5-Sigma)	• Surgeon Preference Card picking accuracy to 4-Sigma (from 1.5-Sigma) • One or more ORs closing earlier in the day • Surgeon block time adjusted to earlier in the day and/or less block time per surgeon • Fewer OR staff hours in the AM before the 1st case starts

Continued

Continued

Core Process	Cost Recovery Goal	Process Translation Goal	Observable Impact
Patient Care Throughput	Top quartile cost per discharge 85% "sweet spot" staffing (versus 70% current)	• 2pm discharge at 4-Sigma (from 1-Sigma [4pm]) • 60-min bed turnover from physician discharge order • 30-min ED request for bed to ED transfer	• Fewer 3pm-11pm and 11pm-7am staff, or • If high patient demand, more admits per 24-hour day per unit • Fewer inpatients being held in ED
Care Management	Top quartile cost per discharge and LOS for top 12 DRGs	• InterQual or EBM criteria at 4-Sigma • Variation in top correlation resource use per DRG at Three Sigma	• Case managers speak more often about their impact on LOS and cost • Higher case load per case manager due to less items to inspect per patient
Revenue Cycle	Top quartile A/R days Top quartile cost per registration	• 1st process "clean claims" / total claims at 90% • USL "days to clean claim billing" at 5 days	• Fewer claim adjudications from 3rd Party Payors • Fewer staff in business office

level, of organizational entities, clinical product lines, and functional levels. This requires the deployment of an organization system map through at least four layers of a typical integrated delivery network (IDN). An example of an acute care facility process map appears in Figure 4.2.

This process map highlights all major core processes within the organization, including admission decision-making, patient care throughput, ED, diagnostic processes, revenue cycle, and so forth. Further, it provides three-year goals for each core process. Finally, we can discern the VP owner of each three-year strategic goal and the Black Belt assigned to aid the VP in accomplishing the goal.

At the IDN level, the importance of process mapping to optimize the effectiveness of Lean-Six Sigma cannot be overstated. The process map will reveal current process redundancies that can be removed as Lean-Six Sigma projects improve process quality yields. For example, one managed care

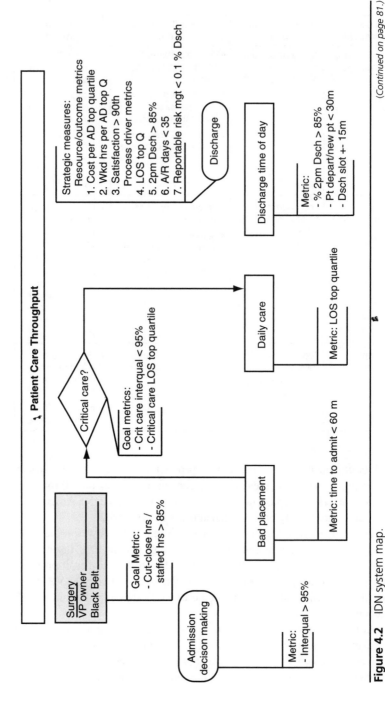

Figure 4.2   IDN system map.

(Continued on page 81.)

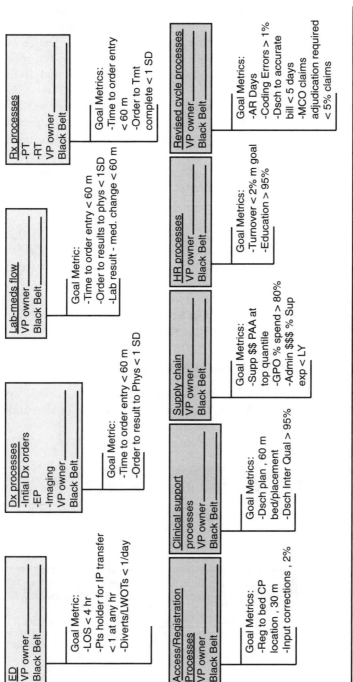

Figure 4.2   IDN system map.

organization was able to reduce 11 redundant FTEs devoted to manual claims adjudication by recognizing the existence of redundancy and then improving quality yields between the medical center and the managed care organization. Without an IDN-level system mapping exercise, this redundancy would never have been observed. Quality was improved 10-fold while recovering almost $500,000 in Cost of Quality costs. These redundancies are very difficult to spot without a system mapping exercise.

Ensuring that the Lean-Six Sigma deployment remains strategic and not a collection of unrelated projects requires that senior leaders link the long-term expectations of the Lean-Six Sigma effort to specific strategic goals; that an organization process map highlight department relationships and redundancies; that project chartering follow a standardized, disciplined process; and that strategic results are diligently tracked to make timely midcourse corrections.

One effective method to develop process maps, created by JCAHO and comprising 50% of the survey process in its Tracer Methodology (Caldwell 2005), is to get a team to physically walk the path of the patient (or any input) throughout the process, interviewing staff along the way and collecting data. The end product is a much more highly refined throughput analysis that uncovers interrelationships, interdependencies, bottlenecks, and hour-by-hour mismatches between capacity, staffing, and demand.

Assign Accountable Executives to Each Core Process

In many cases, the senior leader roles, illustrated in Figure 4.3, exist within the organization. A clinical effectiveness group, for instance, often

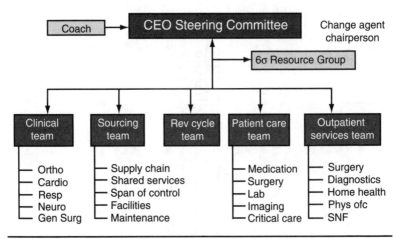

Figure 4.3   Lean-Six Sigma Resource Group.

serves as a clinical team and simply emerges after Lean-Six Sigma deployment with redefined missions. Other roles may not exist at all and consideration must be given to how the roles will be achieved. In smaller organizations, a merger of the CEO Steering Committee and the five core process groups can be considered. It is important to note that the names of these accountable groups are not the critical point—that is, it is not critical that the senior leader oversight group be called the "Steering Committee," but rather that the roles are represented and perform their roles flawlessly.

These four roles exist in most effective infrastructures:

1. CEO Steering Committee

2. Chief strategist

3. Coach

4. Accountable executives

CEO Steering Committee

The main task of the CEO Steering Committee, usually chaired by the chief operating officer or other senior executive in the role of chief strategist of the Lean-Six Sigma initiative, is to ensure that the Lean-Six Sigma effort is strategically deployed, not just a collection of interesting projects. One of the most common pitfalls of Lean-Six Sigma efforts in healthcare is they are decidedly tactical in nature.

The CEO Steering Committee's role includes establishing clear goals for each core process as discussed above, based on available comparative data if available. For example, the Revenue Cycle Team might own the strategic goal to "release 90% clean claims in five days by fiscal year-end," the Patient Care Team's goal might be to "achieve top quartile expense per department statistic in 80% of departments by fiscal year-end," and the Patient Care Throughput Team might work to "achieve 2 P.M. discharge by 95% patients by year-end." These tasks require realized expectations that as teams improve quality, reduce cycle times, and reduce errors, they recapture Cost of Quality, as discussed in Chapter 1.

The second major function of the CEO Steering Committee is to establish and track strategic metrics illustrating movement of critical indicators on the balanced scorecard.

A third major function is to serve as a "learning lab" for senior executives. Executives can sponsor presentation of innovations reported in the literature, peer review journals, conferences, or other forms of education. The sponsoring executive leads the discussion of three topics. What key learnings emerge from this review? What, if any, are the implications for us? What action plan can we launch and which executive will lead it?

Another major function is to aid the accountable executives who make up the Steering Committee in constructing action plans to achieve their goals and to hold the project teams and the managers within them accountable for rapid strategic results as contained in their deployment plans, constantly pushing for speed.

The final major function, in concert with the Lean-Six Sigma Resource Group, is to ensure that the accountable executives select logical projects. Not all projects should be DMAIC efforts. Some are best approached through a 100-Day Workout or a PCDA-type process.

A major weakness of many Lean-Six Sigma programs in healthcare is assuming that Lean-Six Sigma is a single method—DMAIC. This fallacy leads to wasted effort and time. Rather, strategically driven Lean-Six Sigma programs contain multiple methods selected based upon the goal to be attained and the presence or absence of a process-specific solution set from which to rapidly execute.

Chief Strategist

The chief strategist, the chair of the CEO Steering Committee, enjoys the primary duty and privilege of ensuring that the infrastructure achieves the strategic goals critical to the organization's success. Most often this person is the COO, but it can be any senior leader, including the CEO, with the will, knowledge, and skill set to get results.

Coach

The coach, often a person outside the organization, aids the chief strategist, Lean-Six Sigma Resource Group, executive leaders, and project team leaders in constructing, deploying, and redesigning their deployment plans for speed.

Accountable Executives

As mentioned many times up to this point, each core process after having three- to five-year goals established and mapped to the overall organization system map, is assigned to executives who inherit accountability for achieving those strategic results and manage the Lean-Six Sigma Black Belts and project managers engaged in carrying out projects over time.

Deploy a Lean-Six Sigma Resource Group

The main function of the Lean-Six Sigma Resource Group and the infrastructure it manages is to drive results from projects. It has been stated many times in this book that it is not the role of the senior leader team to charter projects and ensure their results project by project. Rather, it is the role of the accountable executive in charge of a core process strategy and the Lean-Six Sigma Resource Group director to ensure project results. Specific groups of people are needed to manage the strategic deployment of Lean-Six Sigma in any organization, and an effective infrastructure includes many roles, each with its own critical functions.

Lean-Six Sigma Resource Group

Figure 4.4 illustrates the relationships of the roles involved in the Lean-Six Sigma infrastructure.

The Resource Group serves two purposes. First, the leader of this group, a Master Black Belt, aids the chief strategist and CEO Steering Committee by managing the infrastructure and, second, the Resource Group houses the organization's Black Belts. While two themes regarding Black Belt reporting structures exist in the field—in some organizations the Black Belts report directly within selected departments and in some they report directly to the director of the Lean-Six Sigma Resource Group—ultimately, the most effective schema is the latter structure. The reason many organizations deploy Black Belts to the department level is that they have been coached by non-healthcare consulting firms to organize in this way. In large manufacturing and service companies, in which large divisions exist, enough Master Black Belts and Black Belts exist to assign a Master Black Belt and several Black Belts to every division (Breyfogle, 2003, 26–27). However, almost no healthcare organization is large enough to staff an adequate number of Master Black Belts and assigned Black Belts to make this structure work.

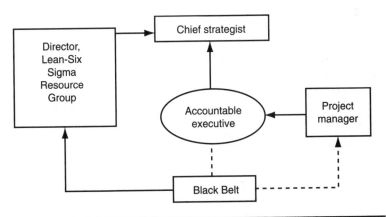

Figure 4.4   Lean-Six Sigma Resource Group relationships.

In most healthcare organizations a typical structure for a manufacturing division will more than adequately staff the entire Lean-Six Sigma initiative. However, a reasonable rule of thumb is that deploying Black Belts throughout the organization would make sense if at least two Master Black Belt groups, made up of at least three Black Belts each, could be deployed under two or more accountable executives. In this case, the structures discussed earlier would be duplicated for each division.

Resource Group Return on Investment. The key metrics for the effectiveness of the Lean-Six Sigma Resource Group are:

- Resource Group return on investment (ROI): Generally, any quality resource group, whether it is the Lean-Six Sigma Resource Group, case managers, quality professionals, medical staff committee analysts, or risk managers, should produce a minimum of 5:1 return on the expenses of the department. In the absence of this ROI, the department can be classified as overhead and according to the evaluation of one northeastern health system CEO, "this is no time to be considered overhead."

- Percent of projects achieving stated goals on time as specified in project charters.

Many Resource Group directors will argue that Black Belts do not control whether or not a manager executes. Many directors of case management will argue that case managers do not control length of stay. The CEO could just as easily assert that she cannot control LOS, but it is highly unlikely that the board would accept this logic. At the end of the day, not someone, but everyone, must be accountable for something and these "somethings" must ultimately drive the organization's key metrics.

Determining the Number of Black Belts Needed. While the most common factor in the dialogue regarding the number of Black Belts needed when discussed among executive leaders is the labor cost involved of adding FTEs to the organization, in the case of Black Belts their cost is not the major factor. As Table 4.2 suggests, the number of Black Belts required should be driven by the following factors:

- How much Cost of Quality recovery is required over the next few years?

- How much cost recovery do we expect the average project to return?

- How many months do we anticipate each project to require?

- How many projects can our core processes manage simultaneously?

These factors determine the formula to calculate the number of fulltime equivalent Black Belts that should make up the Lean-Six Sigma Resource Group.

As Table 4.2 illustrates, for a $10 million COQ recovery goal, five fulltime equivalent Black Belts would be needed, but as the COQ recovery climbs, the number of required projects, and hence the required Black Belts, increases.

Another schema is to determine the number of Black Belts based upon the number of accountable executives on the Steering Committee who will be deploying projects. Generally, one fulltime Black Belt can be shared between two accountable executives. Some executives, such as the chief nursing officer or vice president of patient care, can keep one to two Black Belts fully engaged (that is, patient care throughput is often large enough to accommodate two to four DMAIC projects simultaneously).

Again, the driving factor should not be the number of FTEs added or the cost of the Lean-Six Sigma Resource Group, but rather the number of Black Belts required to get the job done.

Additional Role for Green Belts. Green Belts have less training and experience than Black Belts. While most aggressive and/or complex opportunities require the more skilled Black Belts, many projects are within the

Table 4.2   Determining number of Black Belts.

	$10 million COQ Recovery in 24 months	$20 million COQ Recovery in 24 months
Number of projects required at $250,000 per project (6 months each)	40	80
Number of projects that must run simultaneously to achieve results in 24 months	10	20
Number of fulltime Black Belts at 2 simultaneous projects (4 per year if projects completed in 6 months)	5	10
Results achieved in 24 months if only 2 Black Belts	$1 Million	$1 Million

capabilities of Green Belts. Breyfogle (2003, 28) suggests that, while the traditional path for a Green Belt is to advance to Black Belt, another construct is to use the training resources allocated to roll out the Lean-Six Sigma Resource Group to train a few staff employed in high-leverage departments in Green Belt skills. In this way, Lean-Six Sigma tools and methods can be leveraged throughout the organization. This is particularly helpful for smaller functions such as physicians offices, smaller outpatient functions, and off-site campuses not in the strategic mainstream.

Becoming a Black Belt. While variations around the general theme exist, the Black Belt designation is one of skill demonstration. Any other way of certification signals a kiss of death. Black Belts are not individuals who attend a course, read a book, or earn the designation because they are exceptional analysts or industrial engineers. The Black Belt is determined by pure demonstration of results. And these project results must be defended before a Master Black Belt familiar with the organization's bottom-line needs. Certification can be demonstrated only in this way. In the way of skills, Black Belts must demonstrate intimate knowledge in the use of statistical software, such as MINITAB®, and project management software, such as Microsoft Project. Without demonstrated ability to construct data sets and analyze them in MINITAB® or similar software, one cannot effectively manage a project. There is no other way.

The most common progression begins with Apprentice, a "would-be" Black Belt who observes one DMAIC project and runs through Green Belt and Black Belt to Master Black Belt. An individual earns Green Belt status upon completion of one DMAIC project while under the watchful eye of a Black Belt or Master Black Belt.

Usually, it is best to pair Green Belts to manage one project together, so they can build skill sets together in this first time out in the real world. A Green Belt evolves to Black Belt status by successfully completing a second DMAIC project while aiding a pair of Green Belts, again under the watchful eye of a Black Belt or Master Black Belt. It is not uncommon for Green Belts and Black Belts to repeat a rotation before achieving certification.

A Master Black Belt is an individual who is exceptionally skilled in teaching and coaching statistics and engineering and has succeeded in three or more DMAIC projects. Not all Black Belts become Master Black Belts.

Some organizations find the Black Belt label distasteful and create their own labels. For example, a Florida healthcare system prefers Assistant Coach, Coach, and Head Coach.

Further, it is important to note that the progress does not signify a pecking order or supervisory structure in the usual context of supervision. Instead, these designations are more akin to clinical ladders in nursing in which designations are earned via demonstrated competence.

Black Belts as Full Time or Part Time. The highest ROI will result from having the Black Belts reside within the Resource Group, although some organizations have been successful with Black Belts deployed to individual departments. While some organizations devote full-time staff to the Black Belt roles, many do not. Full-time Black Belts manage two to three DMAIC projects at any given time; therefore, a 0.5 full-time equivalent Black Belt with another 0.5 job could arguably manage one to two DMAIC projects. However, we have observed that under the part-time model, both jobs suffer at inopportune times. For example, at certain times the Black Belt will have vital tasks that must be completed quickly in both roles. It is not likely that the accountable executive will appreciate seeing an ill-prepared Black Belt at a critical meeting with physicians. Nor is it likely that the other manager will be delighted if her report to the CEO is delayed because the Black Belt was consumed with a DMAIC activity. It is a no-win situation and, in the end, the quality of both jobs suffers and the ROI of the Black Belt is suboptimized.

While there are pros and cons around the issue of full-time versus adjunct Black Belts—and assertive proponents of both views make exceptional points in their own favor—the reality is that both approaches have advantages and both have weaknesses. Hence, the debate should be decided by the leaders of the organization on the merits of those pros and cons and their consequences. Each case is different.

Selecting Black Belt Candidates. Black Belts must not only possess the capacity to learn and apply statistical and engineering methods, but also must be able to exert the soft skills so vital in driving change within a work group (Breyfogle 2003, 29–31). However, if a single characteristic must be singled out it would be that a Black Belt is someone *who gets things done.* The two major hard skills are:

- *Statistical and engineering applications*—working with data and process mapping

- *Project management*—bringing results in on time

Project management effectiveness is not present in all great analysts, and statistical and engineering ability is not always present in strong project managers. But, at the end of the day, results can occur only when projects are completed on time. Both skills are vital. The easiest assessment vehicle is to identify individuals who can present several examples of projects they personally completed, including evidence that the analysis was actually performed (that is, they did not delegate analysis to others). And, that they developed and implemented the plans to conclusive, measurable results via demonstrated detailed project plans. Although choosing an individual who merely expresses a strong interest has worked on many occasions, it is very risky business, and failure harms the individual as well as the organization.

While candidates possessing the hard skills exist throughout the organization, logical starting points are existing management or industrial engineers, financial and clinical analysts, information technology, or any other individuals who regularly work with and present complex data. One caveat regarding existing management engineers should be noted. Many organizations have management engineers whose sole function for several years has been the management of comparative financial benchmark data. Many of these management engineers view their roles ending when the data are sent to the department managers and have little appetite or skills for driving change—the so-called soft skills. Executives will be setting these individuals up for failure and disappointment by selecting them as Black Belt apprentices. A strong management engineer or any analyst can continue to provide vital support without having to become a Black Belt. Identifying individuals with soft skills is more problematic. One insightful COO recently observed, "I can't describe the characteristics of someone with strong change management skills, but I can point her out to you as soon as I see her."

Certification of Black Belts. A final observation about progressive skill acquisition. Some organizations attempt to acquire Lean-Six Sigma expertise by sending one or more individuals to a course in which they complete projects and present to the class of outsiders. This is not an effective route to introduce a Lean-Six Sigma competency. While a little more expensive upfront, on-the-ground apprenticing of the first wave of Green Belts is a high predictor of success. It should be a no-brainer, however, to recognize the value of this apprenticing process when leaders understand that each DMAIC project should produce a minimum of $150,000 cost recovery, and up to $500,000 in many projects, in almost any organization. In fact, the CEO, chief strategist, and CEO Steering Committee should set the bar for the Resource Group's return on investment at $150,000 per FTE Black Belt per year in a midsized organization.

Project Leaders and Project Teams

The role of project leaders and their project teams is ultimately to execute. This probably sounds simple, but, as uncovered in the *Good to Great in Healthcare* research (Pieper 2004), one of the biggest differences between quantum improvers and nonstarters is simply the failure to execute. Quantums follow a pattern of plan, implement, implement, implement, while Nonstarters follow plan, plan, plan, plan. . . .

Project Chartering Process

Disciplined use of a standardized project chartering and milestones tracking process was a consistent finding in the *Good to Great in Healthcare* research (Caldwell 2004c). The use of standardized processes, approaches, and chartering documents ensures that all critical factors are considered and promotes learning because managers throughout the organization can gain knowledge from their colleagues without possessing detailed knowledge of the process under improvement. An effective project chartering process contains the following elements:

- Projects are chartered by accountable executives in pursuit of their defined three- to five-year strategic goals, not by the Steering Committee or by department managers.

- Projects are laid out over time to achieve a three- to five-year goal, not selected moment by moment. This project planning structure, called "waves," is illustrated in Figure 4.5. While the specific focus area of a project expected to launch in 12 months might not be known, a broad focus area and anticipated cost recovery can be estimated so that future project activity can be forecast by the accountable executive, project leaders, and Black Belts.

- Multiple project types, as discussed in Chapter 3, are conducted simultaneously based upon the capacity for simultaneous projects within a given core process.

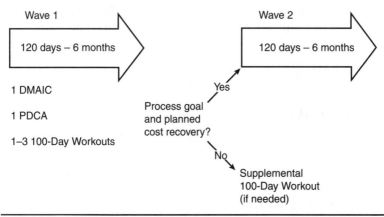

Figure 4.5   Project wave structure.

Large core processes, such as patient care throughput, might sustain two DMAICs, three to five PDCAs, and three to five 100-Day Workouts simultaneously, while smaller core processes, such as ED, might be able to accommodate only one DMAIC and one 100-Day Workout at the same time.

- Each project charter contains a process goal (critical "Y") that, if achieved, will lead to Cost of Quality recovery as the exhaust. This COQ recovery is quantified during the chartering process.

- A detailed project plan is completed by the project leader and Black Belt, highlighting critical time milestones that must be achieved for the project to come in on time and produce the required results to achieve the three- to five-year strategic goal(s).

- A contingency plan is scheduled before the project kickoff, often in the form of a Supplemental 100-Day Workout, in anticipation that the project will fail to meet its chartered cost recovery. The Supplemental 100-Day Workout is canceled when it becomes clear that the project will achieve its cost recovery goal. This construct is most vital. It is a fact of organizational life that not all projects will achieve their objectives. The usual and customary approach is to plan and implement remedial action after the original project's suboptimal results become known. This remedial process, if indeed it occurs at all, requires a significant amount of time to plan, organize, and implement. Wasted time is the enemy of rapid cycle change; therefore, the more effective course of action is to plan and schedule in advance the Supplemental 100-Day Workout as a contingency activity and cancel it if it is not needed.

- Collectively, project charters are reviewed, discussed, and managed by the accountable executives who make up the Steering Committee. As mentioned earlier, a kiss of death for any Lean-Six Sigma deployment is to assign the role of chartering and tracking projects to the Steering Committee, as highlighted in Figure 4.6.

Rather, it is the role of the accountable executives who make up the Steering Committee to work collaboratively to manage the project structure as a Lean-Six Sigma strategy deployment team, as illustrated in Figure 4.7.

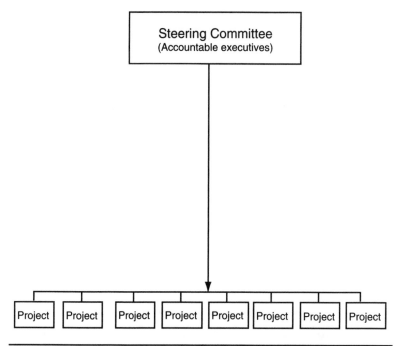

Figure 4.6   Ineffective tactical project approach.

MEASURING STRATEGIC MAGIC MOMENT RESULTS

Deploy a senior leader-driven strategic tracking system that makes success—and the lack of success—highly visible. The result of such a process is diligent midcourse correction if completed projects are failing to achieve the required strategic results. Success of any strategy deployment method, including Lean-Six Sigma, requires extensive pulse checking from time to time. An effective tracking system creates action plans or adjusts existing action plans more than once a year, but not as frequently as quarterly, and certainly not monthly. An annual planning process leaves too much at risk if projects are behind, and quarterly action planning requires too much time to be invested in tracking versus execution. The ideal method is to respond to strategic results every 100 days, while checking on critical project milestones biweekly or monthly. This is not to suggest, of course, that if a disastrous event occurs during a particular month and no action plan exists that

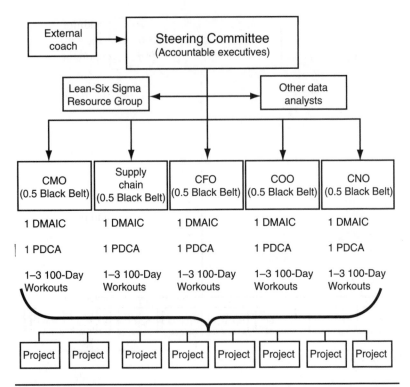

Figure 4.7   Effective strategic project approach.

some action is not warranted; rather, organizations should avoid the tempta-
tion to adjust existing plans after only a month of implementation when new
results appear.

To track strategic results, organizations adopt a number of successful
templates. Some form of balanced scorecard is likely to be found in many
healthcare organizations. When using a balanced scorecard with Lean-Six
Sigma deployment, however, a radical transformation of the strategic mind-
set is required. Instead of tracking average performance, a Lean-Six Sigma
balanced scorecard tracks against the customer "repel" point. For example,
rather than track the average length of stay for an emergency department
patient, Lean-Six Sigma organizations will track the percentage of patients
whose stay is less than 150 minutes, attempting to drive this to the Six
Sigma level, or 99.9997%.

Eight key concepts form the underlying framework of an effective balance scorecarding process. First, not all measures are created equal, and

measuring more often than you intend to act is waste. In addition, budget and thresholds are poor drivers toward world-class performance, you cannot be all things to all people, and one concept is especially important to executives: Without balance, leaders topple.

But the concepts of effective balance scorecarding that are most vital to Lean-Six Sigma deployment are these:

- Form follows function.
- Rate of improvement is the most vital measure for quantum improvement.
- Use leading indicators versus trailing indicators.
- Maintain a line of sight from strategic imperatives and project execution.

1. Form Follows Function

The format of a measurement panel should be driven by what you are trying to achieve. Balanced scorecards typically come in three forms: the spider diagram, the red light–green light table in tabular form, and the strategic run chart when data over time is desirable.

Spider Diagram. The most popular scorecard format is the spider diagram, which is useful for visualizing performance from all dimensions. Spider diagrams can be constructed by using PowerPoint, Excel, Harvard Graphics, and other presentation software. Two factors deserve attention. The first factor is the actual metrics under observation; for instance, cash flow as a percentage of net income, patient satisfaction, or medication errors per 100 case mix adjusted discharge. The second factor is the thresholds of performance.

The underlying concepts of the spider diagram were developed by Noriega Kano of Toyota. Kano recognized, as former GE executive Jack Welch did later, that there are two dimensions of performance—repelling quality, or quality at levels below which customers will defect to competitors, and attractive quality, or quality at levels that sustain return customer loyalty. Case studies by Kano suggested that customer expectations, both repelling quality and attractive quality, do not exhibit along a linear scale but rather along an exponential curve (Kano 1996).

For example, the ED patient loyalty rating does not climb proportionately with the number of minutes spent in the ED. Rather, ED patients are repelled and will walk out without treatment at 250 minutes, but the benefit of declining treatment times levels off at about 120 minutes. That is, there is little customer loyalty gain below 120 minutes. On a spider diagram, the

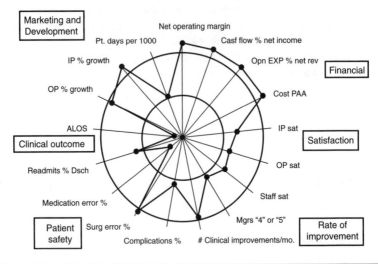

Figure 4.8   Spider diagram.

| | Above stretch | | On target | | Below target |

LAST FY ACTUAL

CURRENT YTD STATUS

MM	Stretch	Actual	MM	Stretch	Status
Customer Satisfaction	83%	Hit stretch	Customer Satisfaction	83%	○
Contribution Margin	160% of budget	Hit stretch	Contribution Margin	105% Budget	■
Revenue	130% of budget	Hit stretch	Revenue	105% Budget	■
Penetrate new markets	10 new market segments	Hit stretch	70% managers achieve "4" or "5"	80%	○
Reduce medication errors 25%	30%	Hit target	Medication errors 25%	30%	○

FY 1Q STATUS

PROPOSED NEXT FY GOALS

MM	Stretch	MM	Stretch
Customer Satisfaction	NM	Customer Satisfaction	83%
Contribution Margin	88%	Contribution Margin	105% of budget
Gross Revenue	85%	Gross Revenue	105% of budget
30% mgrs at "4" or "5"	35%	70% mgrs "4" or "5"	80%
Medication errors 25%	30%	Surgical errors 25%	30%

Figure 4.9   Red light–green light table.

inner and outer circles illustrate these dimensions. The inner circle represents performance below which customers will rebel and, hence, immediate crisis action by senior management is warranted. The outer circle represents that point beyond which high customer loyalty is achieved.

Red Light–Green Light Table. The red light–green light table was popularized by Larry Abramson while a senior vice president at Premier, Inc. This visual control has the additional feature of viewing past and current performance, along with future thresholds. Because of this feature and its ease of interpretation, the red light–green light table has become a preferred balanced scorecard for many people.

Strategic Run Chart. There are times when it is desirable to view performance over time, instead of a snapshot in time, with a perspective toward future performance expectations. In this case, the strategic run chart is the best medium. An analogy might be the difference between a photo album and a movie. If strategic run charts are used extensively and senior management maintains 16 strategic measures, several pages will be required, which is its only real downside. Some leaders choose to use the red light–green light table and the strategic run charts simultaneously, viewing just the top two or three strategic measures on the run charts.

2. Rate of Improvement

The second key concept of balanced scorecarding relevant to Lean-Six Sigma deployment is the importance of improving the rate of improvement. All balanced scorecards, regardless of format, contain categories of measures. At a minimum, the following is observed:

- Financial
- Customer satisfaction
- Clinical outcome
- Marketing
- Patient safety

However, a performance dimension that is often overlooked is the rate of improvement, or how quickly the organization executes new ideas. If a CEO can have only one measure, that measure should be the rate of improvement. In support of this argument, the Baldrige National Quality Award criteria weightings were adjusted recently to include heavy emphasis on diffusion of innovation.

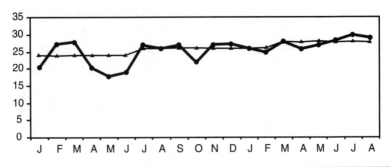

Figure 4.10   Strategic run chart.

So, if measuring rate of improvement is vital to a balanced scorecard, how might it be measured? While there are many approaches to this dimension of performance, a simple measure is the number of days from project kickoff until execution. Some argue that the magnitude of the change is important to measure, but because magnitude is covered in the other dimensions, measuring it here is not necessary. In doing so, a stretch goal can be set to decrease the number of days per project by 20% per year. Over time, the continually decreasing project cycle time would double the number of completed projects per year.

3. Leading Indicators versus Trailing Indicators

The importance of leading indicators over trailing indicators is another key concept of balanced scorecarding relevant to Lean-Six Sigma deployment. David Luther, who headed Corning's quality effort during the 1980s and early 1990s and is a leading thinker in the field of performance measurement, observed that by the time market-share increases (or decreases) were detected, too much time had passed between the strategic interventions and the measurement. Therefore, organizations are best served by tracking proxy measures that are more real-time than trailing.

For example, instead of market share, track the percent increase in net income versus the past 12 months. This rolling month-to-month indicator has the advantage of picking up changes rapidly. Or, in addition to patient satisfaction, which in some organizations trails the patient's experience by six months or more, track the number of complaints per 100 adjusted discharges. Of course, this is not to suggest ignoring key trailing indicators. Instead, the performance tracking should focus on leading indicators that are then validated retrospectively as trailing indicators become available.

4. Line of Sight from Strategies to Project Execution

The final key concept of balanced scorecarding relevant to Lean-Six Sigma deployment is the notion that all projects should be linked directly to a strategic priority. All organizations possess a finite capacity for improvement work. There are only so many Black Belts, and each can manage only about two to four projects simultaneously. Managers have only so many hours per week to devote to improvement work. Hence, the importance of selecting the right projects is vital to success.

Dr. Joseph Juran coined a phrase to express this phenomenon—"necessary and sufficient." That is, are all chartered projects necessary to achieve the strategy or have a few nonstrategic projects crept in? If all projects achieve the intended results and come in on time, are they sufficient to achieve the strategy? That's why it is vitally important to have a line of sight between Lean-Six Sigma projects and the key strategies of an organization. A helpful tool to illustrate our project alignment is the strategy deployment tree shown in Figure 4.11.

Readers interested in leading a discussion with senior leaders can find an electronic version of the described discussion on the CD. (Instructions are found at the end of this chapter.)

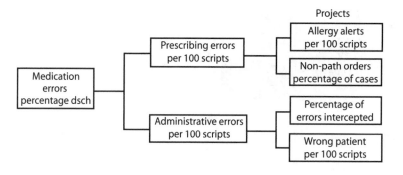

Figure 4.11   Strategy deployment tree diagram.

ESTABLISH MONTHLY PROJECT MILESTONE TRACKING

An important factor uncovered in the *Good to Great in Healthcare* research (Pieper 2004) was that quantum improvers followed a disciplined tracking process to detect as early as possible that a project's goals would not be met.

The specific form of tracking varied from sophisticated, intranet-based, milestone tracking to "back of the napkin" approaches. So, it is not the sophistication of the tracking process that makes the difference, but rather that the chosen process is used consistently and in the same form throughout the organization. While there are many tracking tools, such as Microsoft Project, homegrown tools using Excel, Word, or other software will suffice. The importance is that it is done. Web-based tools, such as EXCELerator™ at www.chipcaldwellassoc.com, automate this tracking process, saving manager time for the more important tasks of implementation. Figures 4.12 and 4.13 illustrate an effective tracking tool used in the Operations Waste 100-Day Workout. The patient care division roll-up provides real-time monthly feedback regarding the collective impact of all division managers' planned and actual implementation against the Operations Waste 100-Day Workout target.

Figure 4.13 represents one manager's detail plan containing the above patient care division roll-up from EXCELerator.™

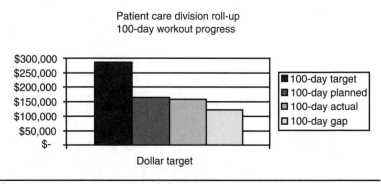

Figure 4.12   EXCELerator™ Web-based automated tracking system.

SENIOR LEADER MISSTEPS

When asked to describe their Lean-Six Sigma initiatives, many organizations deploying Six Sigma describe their programs as a set of projects at the department level. The imaging department did this, the surgery department did that. From a senior executive perspective, this appears strategically disorganized and a bit like anarchy. Listening to the executive, manager, or Black Belt describe these projects sounds like the organization is simply executing a sequential series of unrelated projects and no discernable strat-

Memorial Medical

Lean-Six Sigma 100-Day Workout Action Plan

	Dollar Target	FTET Target
FY05 Target	$ 330,380	3.87
100-Day Target	$ 132,152	1.55
100-Day Planned	$ 3,333	
100-Day Actual	$ 3,333	
100-Day Gap	$ 128,820	
FY05 Gap	$ 327,048	

Funct. Area	In-patient Services
Leader	Tom Barkram
Admin Director	Joan Gibbs
Dept.	Pharmacy

FY04 Cycles:

1st 100-Day Window: Oct 21–Feb 1; Report-out 2/11
2nd 100-Day Window: Feb 11–May 30; Report-out TBD
3rd 100-Day Window: Jun 15–sep 30; Report-out TBD

Item #	Cost Center	Actions Subaccount description and action to be taken	Due Date	Actual Date	Validation date	Comparison FY04 Actual Dollars	Comparison FY05 Budget Dollars	Savings (Annualized) 1st 100-Day	2nd 100-Day	3rd 100-Day	FY Total	100-Day Actual
1	7710	Change pharmacy closing time to 11pm, elim 1 PHam FTE	2/1	2/1	2/1	$ 179,000	$ –	$ 132,152	$ 132,152	$ 132,152	$ 396,456	
2	7710	Outsource pharmacist review required by JCAHO standard MM 4.10.1	3/1	3/1	4/1				$ 48,591		$ 48,591	$ –
3	7710	Consolidate RPh coverage between depts vs OT	5/1	5/1	6/1				$ 2,700	$ 127,980	$ 127,980	$ –
4	7710	Consolidate 2 part-time into 1 FT posn	7/1	7/15	9/15			$ 3,333			$ 2,700	$ –
5											$ 3,333	$ 3,333
6											$ –	$ –
		Total				$ 179,000	$ –	$ 3,333	$ 51,291	$ 127,980	$ 182,604	$ 3,333

Figure 4.13   Patient care division roll-up from EXCELerator.™

egy seems to emerge. If department managers determine their own priorities for project selection, without being highly integrated into a strategic "puzzle," then the massive effort to deploy Lean-Six Sigma projects results in such dilution that it is impossible to achieve any one strategic aim. Instead, one department focuses on process goals that have the effect of improving patient satisfaction, another focuses on process goals that improve inter-department dissatisfiers, and another focuses on process goals that achieve cost recovery. The result at the department level looks cohesive, but at the organization level, it reveals chaos of intent.

In other words, two Lean-Six Sigma project deployment approaches might be observed. One method, often recommended in leading lean thinking or Six Sigma textbooks, is for the executive team to select a group of projects every six months based on the current issues. So, we might see the leadership, in a routine meeting, decide that in this next wave of projects, they will embark upon improving blood ordering in the emergency department, charting time of lab reports, errors in managed care claims, and late start times in surgery. As these projects are completed, they once again examine the issues of the moment and select the next wave of projects that might be totally unrelated to the last wave of projects. Over time, this moment-by-moment approach produces no real, sustainable value to the strategic imperatives pressing upon the organization. Rather, the approach is merely a sophisticated form of putting out fires.

An alternative approach, used by a second organization, might begin with the senior leaders determining that in three years they wished to achieve national benchmark status in medication errors, surgery cost per case, ED LOS, and noon discharge on inpatient units. The vice presidents responsible for these specific core business processes, after examining baseline data, can determine a series of sequential projects that must be accomplished over the next three years to achieve the strategic results desired. The Process Translation Workpaper found in Table 4.1 can serve as an excellent discussion guide to this approach for executive-level planning and learning purposes.

One way to test for the presence of a strategically driven Lean-Six Sigma program is to list the last 10 projects and see if the organization's strategic priorities are evident. If no more than two critical goal types are obvious, then the Lean-Six Sigma effort can be said to be strategic; on the other hand, if there are 10 different aims, then the assumption is that individual managers have been given little guidance in project selection.

Project team presentations to executive management should avoid reviewing why a specific method was deployed or what robust statistical methods were contained in effective Lean-Six Sigma projects. Rather, the presentations should compare baseline data to the new, higher state of process performance. A kiss of death for a Lean-Six Sigma deployment is to begin with discussions of project selection, Black Belt apprenticing, and resource allocation.

SUMMARY

Seven nondelegable senior leader tasks must come together flawlessly to ensure that the organization's Lean-Six Sigma deployment begins and remains strategic, as opposed to tactical, as follows:

- Clearly articulate the strategic aims of the Lean-Six Sigma effort as it relates to the long-term vision and three- to five-year goals, at the IDN, organization, and core process levels.

- Translate core process cost recovery goals into process goals as a basis for Lean-Six Sigma project determination.

- Create and maintain an organization system map highlighting the interrelationships between core functional processes within the organization and their specific three- to five-year goals aimed at achieving the organization's overall three- to five-year goals.

- Assign key accountable executives to each core functional process who create and implement internal metrics, charter Lean-Six Sigma project teams, appoint project leaders and Black Belts to ensure rapid implementation of identified, high leverage process improvements, and adjust plans according to progress toward the three- to five-year goals.

- Deploy a Lean-Six Sigma Resource Group to manage the necessary infrastructure and project schedule to carry out those aims.

- Measure progress toward three- to five-year strategic results using advanced techniques like the balanced scorecard or other measurement template.

- Aggressively track project milestones that have been commissioned by executive leaders to achieve the strategic goals.

CHECKLISTS AND TOOLS
ACCESSIBLE ELECTRONICALLY

- Magic Moment spreadsheet planner—electronic version on the CD.
- Cost Goal to Process Goal Translation Example—electronic version on the CD.
- CEO Role in Lean-Six Sigma Deployments—electronic version on the CD.

RECOMMENDED LEARNING SESSION

Learning Session for a One-Hour Senior Leader Meeting

One member of the executive team should serve as the recorder, capturing feedback on a flipchart. Using the Translation Workpaper from Table 4.1 (or the template on the CD), the executive team should discuss the following questions:

1. For each cost recovery goal listed in column 2, how will improving the process translation goal in column 3 aid in producing cost recovery as exhaust?

2. Which process translations (column 3) are Type 1 direct Cost of Quality recovery focus areas? Type 2 and Type 3 indirect cost recovery? (Review Chapter 2 for descriptions of Type 1, 2, and 3 costs.)

3. What additional project activities must be undertaken to convert those Type 2 and Type 3 indirect costs into hard bottom-line cost recovery results?

REFERENCES

Barry, Robert, Amy C. Murcko, and Clifford E. Brubaker. 2004. *The Six Sigma Book for Healthcare: Improving Outcomes by Reducing Errors.* Chicago: Health Administration Press.

Breyfogle, Forrest. 2003. *Implementing Six Sigma,* 2nd edition. Hoboken, NJ: John Wiley & Sons.

Caldwell, Chip. 1996. *Mentoring Strategic Change.* Milwaukee: ASQ Quality Press.

————. 2004. "Good to Great in Healthcare: A Research Initiative." Conference presented by the American College of Healthcare Executives, St. Louis, May 26, 2004.

————. Interview with Carol Gilhooley, JCAHO Director of Survey Methods Development, February 4, 2005.

Caldwell, Chip, and James Brexler. 2004. "Improving Throughput and Costs Using Lean-Six Sigma." Conference presented by the American College of Healthcare Executives, Key West, FL, January 12–13, 2004.

Caldwell, Chip, and Bruce Tilley. 2004. "Aggressive Cost Reduction Using Lean-Six Sigma." National teleconference presented by the VHA and the American College of Healthcare Executives, Dallas, March 25, 2004.

Healthcare Advisory Board. 1999. *The Clockwork ED.* Washington: Advisory Board Company.

Kano, N., N. Seraku, F. Takahashi, and S. Tsuji. 1996. "Attractive quality and must-be quality." In *The Best on Quality,* edited by John D. Hromi. Vol. 7, Book Series of the International Academy for Quality. Milwaukee: ASQ Quality Press.

Langley, Gerald, Kevin Nolan, Thomas Nolan, Clifford Norman, and Lloyd Provost. 1996. *The Improvement Guide.* San Franciso: Jossey-Bass Publishers.

Pande, Peter, Robert Neuman, and Roland Cavanagh. 2000. *The Six Sigma Way.* New York: McGraw Hill.

Pieper, Shannon. 2004. "Good to Great in Healthcare." *Healthcare Executive.* Chicago: Health Administration Press, 19(3): 21–26.

Pyzdek, Thomas. 2001. *The Six Sigma Handbook.* New York: McGraw Hill.

ADDITIONAL READING

Good to Great in Healthcare Research—16 Disciplines of Quantum Improvers. Pieper, Shannon. 2004. "Good to Great in Healthcare," *Healthcare Executive.* Chicago: Health Administration Press, *19* (3): 21-26.Access on the CD.

Chief Strategist and Accountable Executives as Change Agents. Pyzdek, 49–82, 31-48.

Assessing Organizational Readiness and Determining Key Strategies for Lean-Six Sigma Deployment. Pande, 83–115.

Key Roles for Accountable Executives, Black Belts and Project Managers. Pande, 117–152.

Training and External Coaching Considerations. Pyzdek, 83–131

5

The Role of Senior Leaders: Simulation, Experimentation, and the Cost of Not Getting It Right the First Time

with David M. Ferrin

"Results? Why man, I have gotten lots of results.
I know several thousand things that won't work!"

Thomas Edison

In this chapter we present a process for understanding the value proposition for change for those times of life when it has to be right the first time. In Lean-Six Sigma, designing new systems is a demanding and uncertain process. Robust Lean-Six Sigma simulation is the tool of choice and builds confidence that proposed systems will deliver the operational and financial outcomes promised. It is the best tool, often the only tool, for optimizing throughput, for identifying which benchmark processes should be implemented, and for designing a new facility.

This chapter shows how to test solutions before implementation, finding designs that deliver the greatest value and mitigate risk over time. Through Lean-Six Sigma simulation, one can design robust processes and identify the capacity needed to deliver the value you desire for your operations, staff, and patients.

Modeling processes helps the leader understand the following questions:

- What if implemented changes are not enough?
- What if it is too much or inefficiently deployed?
- How will the new processes perform?
- What risks can be mitigated before implementation?
- Will changes lead in the right direction now and in the future?
- What if the recommended changes could be modeled to show the effects of change before the change is made?

Lean-Six Sigma simulation is a powerful technique used to:

- Prototype and validate business cases and contractual obligations by creating a dynamic model of existing or proposed processes, evaluating the characteristics and behavior of those processes under various operating conditions by simulating demand for those processes.
- Mitigate process performance risk through experimentation with new processes before building and implementing them.
- Assess process sensitivity by understanding how various activities within processes interact and how changes will affect overall performance.
- Promote group understanding, decision making, and buy-in through the use of rigorous analysis and the compelling animation of a dynamic process model.

Lean-Six Sigma simulation addresses:

- How well will our designs perform and how much value can we expect them to deliver?
- What are the bottlenecks and constraints that limit process performance, such as human resources and facility constraints?
- How will our designs perform under different operating scenarios?
- Are our designs pragmatic and implementable?
- Which design alternative will deliver the greatest value (return on investment)?
- How do our designs compare to the current process?

As Figure 5.1 shows, the process of Lean-Six Sigma simulation allows us to balance staffing/resources, process performance, and customer experience.

Through this process we:

- Experiment with process design on the computer, not with people, systems, customers, or investors' money.

- Understand process dynamics: Relate "what it is" to "how it works."

- Use quality animation to accelerate executive understanding and buy-in.

- Build high-confidence process designs so we "don't bet the ranch" on average costs and guesses.

Following are two recent case studies using Lean-Six Sigma simulation in an emergency department and an operating room.

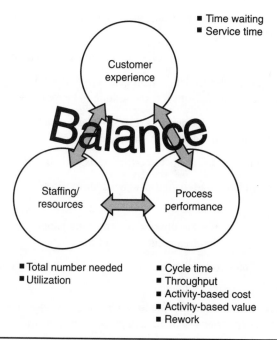

Figure 5.1   Balancing customer demands.

EMERGENCY DEPARTMENT CASE STUDY

A large hospital in the southeastern United States wanted to implement major changes in its main emergency department (ED). The current ED length of stay (LOS) for patients was unacceptably long. The hospital wanted to achieve world-class performance. The objective of this project was to determine the list of available benchmark processes that would yield the best value.

Numerous improvement ideas were proposed. The most promising ideas needed detailed analysis due to the inherent risk associated with patient care. These ideas became Lean-Six Sigma simulation scenarios. The Lean-Six Sigma simulation provided quantifiable performance data that provided input to executive decision making.

Some reasons it takes so long just to get into an ED bed (Advisory Board 1998):

- Large volume of patients in the ED.

- Sicker people are seen first.

- More stable patients are seen first come, first served.

- Both a triage nurse and triage physician must see each patient to assess priority.

- Patient illness requires special rooms with special equipment.

The emergency department's main goal is to find out what's causing the patient problem. Some reasons it takes so long to get out of the ED are:

- ED physicians order multiple tests, such as blood tests, EKG, or x-rays to help diagnose the problem.

- Sometimes it takes hours to perform tests.

- ED physicians need to consult specialists to diagnose the problem.

- ED physicians need to observe patients long enough to determine whether treatments are working.

- It takes hours to admit patients or transfer them to another care facility.

    This project reviewed and identified problem areas with patient flow, patient arrival, department policies, and procedures. Specific areas of investigation included:

- How much will discharging inpatients earlier affect ED LOS?

- Will an additional 30 inpatient beds relieve the ED patient backlog?

- How much bigger should the transitional stay unit (TSU) be to have an effect on ED LOS?

- How many minutes do we need to reduce lab test turnaround time to significantly affect overall patient LOS?

The conceptual model phase included the creation of process maps and documentation. Occasionally, process maps enlighten the client because they typically have never seen their processes modeled end-to-end. They tend to only know fragments of the process and are unaware of the relationship between what they do and the total process outcome. The conceptual model was documented with Microsoft Visio (see Figure 5.2). The model included trigger objects to show patient arrival. It also showed activities, which describe inputs, outputs, required resources, activity durations, and business rules. Finally, the model included decision points for routing patients and objects to show the end of the process.

The programming phase included coding the process model into appropriate simulation software. For this project, Extend by Imagine That was chosen because of its capabilities and affordability. Figure 5.3 illustrates a

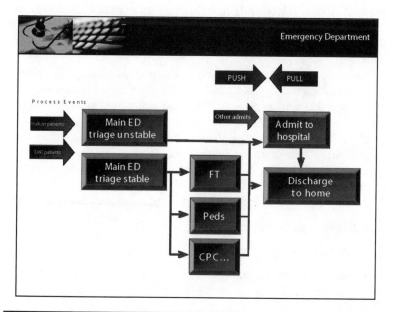

Figure 5.2 Emergency department high-level flowchart.

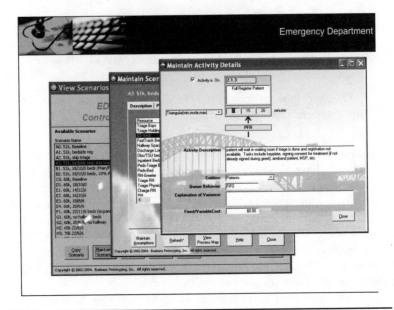

Figure 5.3 Control panel (graphical user interface).

graphical user interface, or control panel, which was developed using Microsoft Access to efficiently manage input parameters to the ED Lean-Six Sigma simulation. For example, the baseline scenario can be copied with the click of a button and input parameters can be changed for a new scenario.

Animation was developed directly in Extend, using hierarchical blocks and bit maps (Figures 5.4 and 5.5). This Lean-Six Sigma simulation used actual hospital layouts as a background, and entity movement and queues were animated on top of the layouts.

The experimentation phase included development of specific scenarios to test. Some of these scenarios required only small changes to data, such as turnaround time for lab or radiology. Other scenarios required more extensive coding changes.

A sampling of the emergency department scenarios evaluated include:

- Baseline (current, as is)

- Inpatient discharge time of day

- Additional inpatient beds

- Additional ED beds

- Surge capacity

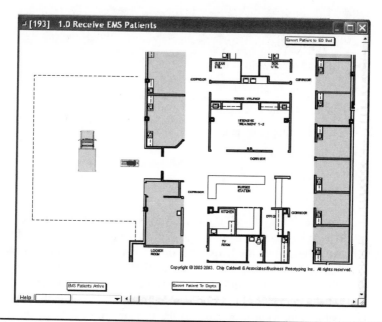

Figure 5.4 Ambulance entrance.

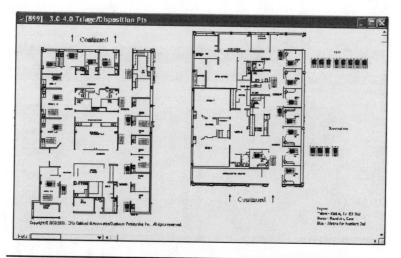

Figure 5.5 Main emergency department.

- Fast track

- Chest pain clinic

- TSU and observation units

- Operational improvements

- Laboratory improvements

- Radiology improvements

- Bedside registration

- Physician triage

- Skipping triage

Discharge time of day (DTOD) analysis is often a strong, value-added scenario for many facilities. Figure 5.6 depicts the basic philosophy of this alternative. The current discharge time of day is determined through analysis of the hospital's inpatient admitting, discharge, and transfer (ADT) information system. This information is profiled by hour of the day, as noted by the lighter bars. The future state, or to-be scenario, signified by the darker bars, is determined relating to the benchmark of 50% of the discharged patients being discharged by 11 A.M. or noon. This is generally a rather difficult initiative to achieve, primarily because significant change is needed to meet the benchmark. For example, physicians need to change rounding processes; case managers and hospitalists must execute their

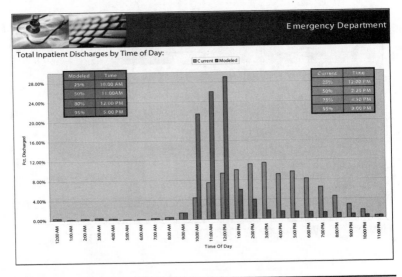

Figure 5.6   Discharge time of day, current and future.

efforts flawlessly; and inpatient support functions, such as housekeeping and transport, must follow suit.

Once implemented, the outcomes are usually very significant, with hospitals realizing between 5% and 15% additional capacity through mostly sunk costs. Moreover, identifying the true value proposition for this initiative is, for all practical purposes, impossible without the use of a valid Lean-Six Sigma simulation. Other approaches are statistically inaccurate and can be very misleading, if not totally off the mark. Studies show that less sophisticated analysis, such as the use of spreadsheets in analyzing simple process impacts, with minor variation can be off as much as 500–600% (Grabau 2001).

Results

After implementation of numerous improvements, the Lean-Six Sigma simulation showed a reduction of 37% in the number of ED patients waiting in the ED for an inpatient bed (Figure 5.7). This is an outstanding result with significant impact on ED patient satisfaction as well as inpatient satisfaction. From a patient throughput perspective, this outcome shows positive influence in the hospital as well as on the support functions.

It is worthy of note that the JCAHO throughput standard (LD 315) looks explicitly for evidence that senior leaders understand boarder patient processes and actively manage to ensure quality care (Caldwell 2005).

Other outcomes of significant note in the ED length of stay are shown in Figure 5.8. Option 1, discharge time of day 50% by noon, reduced ED

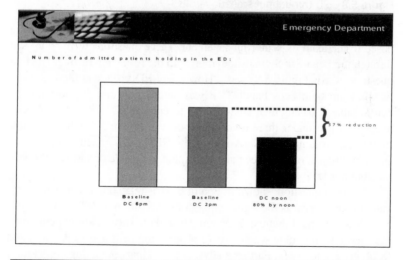

Figure 5.7 Number of ED patients holding for an inpatient bed.

LOS 51%. Option 2, adding an additional 30 inpatient beds, improved ED LOS up to 63%. Option 3, improving ED operations 10%, improved ED LOS 39%. Of course, these improvements are not additive in their impact. It is necessary to evaluate combinations of options independently. Combining options 1 and 2 yields an improvement of 65% in the ED LOS. Combining options 1, 2, and 3 yields an improvement of 72% in the ED LOS.

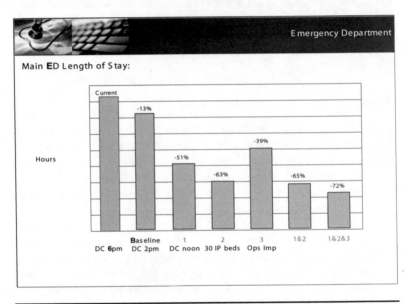

Figure 5.8   ED throughput scenario results.

After the presentation of these results, a number of questions were posed to the team by senior management. These questions were addressed through the Lean-Six Sigma simulation with the following results. The first question asked (Figure 5.9) was, "How many ED visits can the hospital's licensed inpatient beds handle?" It was determined that the hospital felt comfortable in basing their answer upon its current ED LOS, which was an average of just under three hours. As shown in Figure 5.8, when an additional visit volume of 15% is added, the ED LOS jumped dramatically. From Figure 5.9, one can see that the hospital is capable of adding 10% volume but not 15%.

The next question, shown in Figure 5.10, is related to the use of observation beds:" What is the right number of observation beds?" From Figure 5.10, it was learned that the diversion rate and the leave without being seen rates more than double when 6 or 12 observation beds are used, compared to 24 observation beds. Further analysis showed that combining observation beds with a transitional stay unit in a 24-bed unit yielded excellent results.

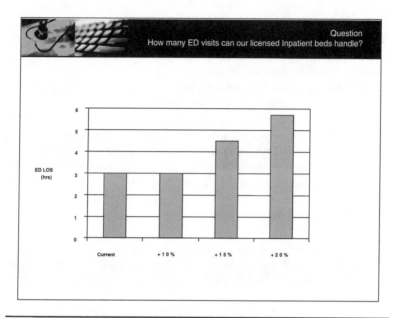

Figure 5.9 How many ED visits can we handle?

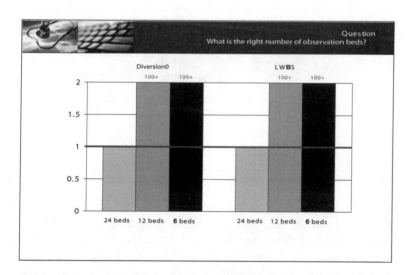

Figure 5.10 What is the right number of observation beds?

Generally speaking, observation beds are used for patients with less than 24 hours inpatient length of stay. A TSU is used primarily to decompress the ED, moving into the TSU the patients who normally wait in an ED for an inpatient bed to become available.

The next question addressed the impact of a discharge lounge. Figure 5.11 identifies the impact through three indicators. This information shows that a six-bed discharge lounge yields a 30% reduction in the percentage of time the ED is full, a 13% improvement in diversion, and a 58% improvement in the leave without being seen rate. This discharge lounge would be only for ED patients being discharged to home in the last 30–45 minutes of their ED visit and who were waiting for test results. The main issue is to monitor them to ensure that they don't decompensate. This option kicks in only when the ED is at least 85% full.

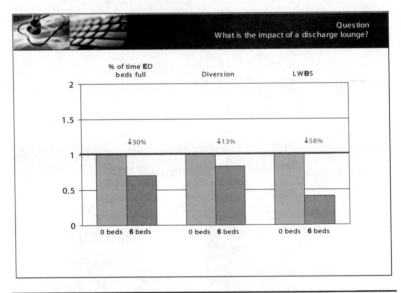

Figure 5.11 What is the impact of the discharge lounge?

The final two questions were concerned with finding the right number of inpatient and ED beds associated with a specific volume of 70,000 ED visits. Figure 5.12 shows that the current inpatients bed count plus 50–80 beds will enable the ED to maintain its current ED LOS. This amount of beds is above the current licensed bed count for the hospital. Consequently, the facility will need to either go through a Certificate of Need (CON) process or somehow constrain the ED below 70,000 annual visits. Figure 5.13 shows that the current number of ED beds plus 9–10 beds will handle the required volume of patients.

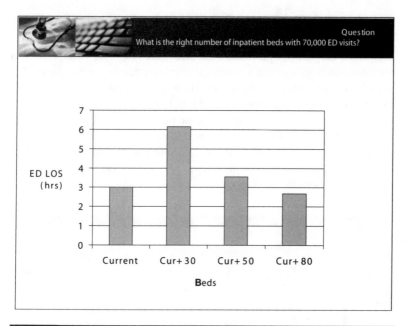

Figure 5.12 What is the right number of inpatient beds with 70,000 ED visits?

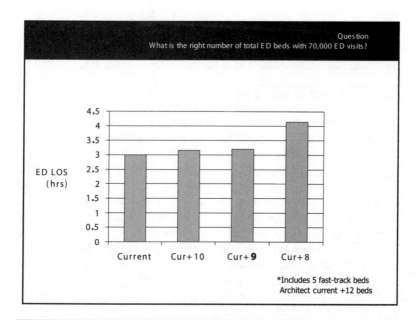

Figure 5.13 What is the right number of ED beds with 70,000 ED visits?

OPERATING ROOM CASE STUDY

Like the emergency department case study, the operating room Lean-Six Sigma simulation also has a graphical user interface or control panel. The associated data requirements, referred to as the data inventory, are roughly two or three times that needed for the ED. The conceptual model (flowchart) is significantly more complex as well because of the complexity encountered in the business rules needed to navigate the OR.

For this project, Extend software was also chosen because of its capabilities and affordability. The animations are based upon actual floor plans for the institution (Figure 5.14).

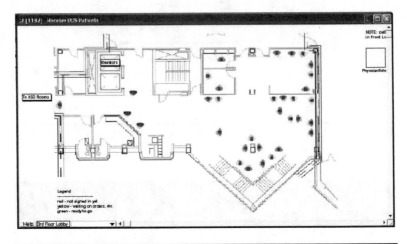

Figure 5.14   Ambulatory surgery department lobby.

Before the day of surgery, pre-admission testing is done to ensure that all test and insurance issues are taken care of before the patient shows up. Although modeled, the animation of that area is not shown here.

Figure 5.14 shows the first entry point during the day of surgery for patients and their guests, the ambulatory surgery department (ASD) or same-day surgery. At this point all patients are checked by registration to ensure that all necessary tests, histories, and physicals are performed as well as insurance and demographic information obtained.

Patients are then escorted to their private ASD rooms, where they are prepared for their procedure (Figure 5.15). Patients return to these rooms upon completion of their procedure in the OR. The use of these rooms is monitored, and an identical fourth-floor unit is used for the same function as well.

From the ASD, patients are moved to OR holding rooms (not shown but animated), where final staging occurs before the patient is moved to the OR

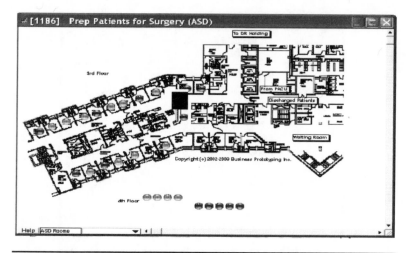

Figure 5.15 ASD room (pre-procedure, post-procedure).

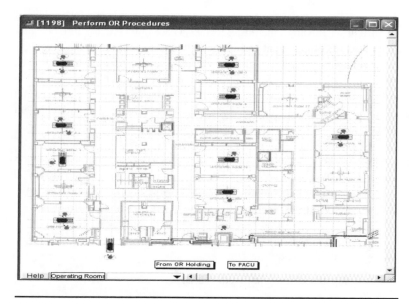

Figure 5.16 Operating rooms.

itself (Figure 5.16). Procedure time is specific to the procedure and the specific physician doing the procedure. Procedure setup and cleanup times are also specific to the procedure, as are the volume and frequency of the procedures. Block schedules are a variable available for evaluation while running scenarios.

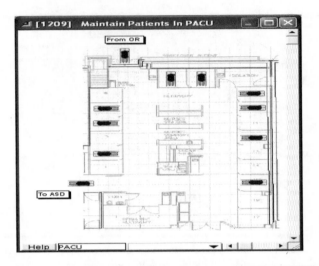

Figure 5.17   Post-anesthesia care unit.

Figure 5.17 shows the post-anesthesia care unit (PACU). PACU acuity is tracked for each patient and is specific to each procedure. Resource use depends upon this acuity, as does the total length of stay in the PACU. After the patients are recovered in the PACU, they are moved back to the ASD to finish their recovery. After staying in the ASD a prescribed amount of time, the patient is either discharged to home or admitted to an inpatient unit.

After all associated information is input into the model and stored through the control panel, a number of scenarios can be run. As is always good practice and methodology, a baseline is established against which all other scenarios are compared. The first baseline is often established using the current operations. Some of the scenarios evaluated are as follows:

- Case cart completion improvement.

- Pre-admission testing done 99%.

- Setup and cleanup time reduced 20%.

- Number of ASD rooms

  - Increased to evaluate the impact on the OR.

  - Reduced to increase the availability of inpatient beds.

- Optimal number of operating rooms.

- Number of pre-op holding bays.

- Number of PACU beds.

- Changes in physician block scheduling.

- Impact of different operational changes on the first surgery case of the day.

- Incentive systems impacts.

- Increased volume by physician group.

- Impact of adding surgical specialties.

- OR utilization studies.

Of course, numerous other scenarios can be investigated. One is limited only by the availability of data, the logic imbedded in the model, time (and money), and one's imagination.

Results

Only a few results will be given. Figure 5.18 shows the impact of improving the OR case cart completion rate from 85% to 99%. This scenario resulted in only a 3% improvement in the cycle time from when the OR called the

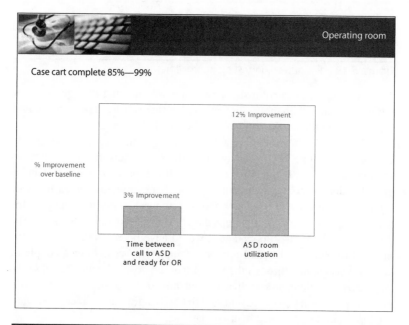

Figure 5.18 OR case cart improvement results.

ASD until the ASD was ready for the OR. More importantly, this scenario resulted in a 12% improvement in the ASD room use, which is significant in regard to the number of staff and rooms needed in the ASD to accommodate the associated OR volume.

Figure 5.19 shows the scenario of improving pre-admission testing (PAT) to essentially 100% of all OR patients. This scenario yields a 5.5% improvement in the on-time starts in the OR and essentially no improvement in the cycle time from when the OR called the ASD until the patient was ready for the OR.

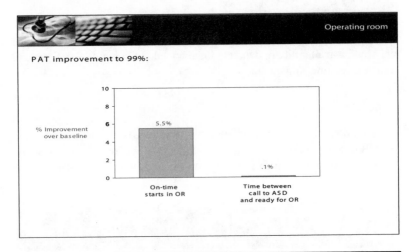

Figure 5.19   Pre-admission testing improvement.

This impact is fairly insignificant and would bring into question the return associated with this improvement. In other words, improving the PAT compliance in this institution may not be worth the effort.

Figure 5.20 shows the impact of improving the procedure setup and cleanup cycle time by 20%. Note that these key performance indicators change only 1–2%. In the grand scheme of life, this is not significant and is probably due to variation within the system. In other words, increasing ASD room has no impact or does no good. A few weeks after this analysis, the team was asked to analyze the impact on the OR of reducing ASD beds. The ASD had beds on two floors, and it would have been advantageous to the hospital to increase the total number of inpatient beds. After a couple of days, it was learned through the model that the hospital could decrease the ASD bed complement significantly but not to the desired extent of one entire unit. Closing an entire unit of ASD beds significantly increased waiting times and total worked hours in the OR.

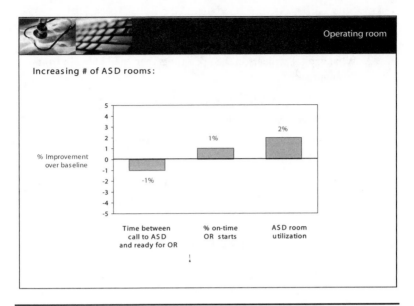

Figure 5.20   Increasing number of ASD rooms has no impact.

SUMMARY

Lean-Six Sigma simulation has proven itself as a valuable addition in the Lean-Six Sigma suite of tools. Moreover, it is often the only tool capable of delivering robust analysis needed for highly complex questions. The strength of the Lean-Six Sigma simulation is its ability to significantly increase the confidence of decision makers in system-related issues, whether they are new facility-related, capacity issues or the value proposition regarding adoption of benchmarked practices. As Edison stated, "Results? Why man, I have gotten lots of results. I know several thousand things that won't work!" Only this way will we find out how well our "improvements" will really work.

RECOMMENDED LEARNING SESSION

Learning Session for a One-Hour Senior Leader Meeting

1. When in the last year would Lean-Six Sigma simulation have helped get buy-in for a project or process?

2. When in the last year did we need more confidence in our decision?

3. What capital projects in the upcoming year would benefit from this approach?

4. For which high-visibility projects during the next year do we expect to use considerable political or financial capital?

5. In which upcoming projects can we not afford a mistake in planning?

6. Would we benefit from a 5–15% improvement in our capacity?

REFERENCES

Caldwell, Chip. 2005. Interview with Carol Gilhooley, JCAHO Director of Survey Methods Development, February 4, 2005.

Clinical Initiatives Center. 1998. *Emergency Care Reform.* Washington, DC: Advisory Board Company.

Ferrin, David, Martin Miller, and Jill Szyzmanski. 2003. *Simulating Six Sigma Improvement Ideas for a Hospital Emergency Department.* Proceedings of the 2003 Winter Simulation Conference, New Orleans.

Grabau, Ken. 2001. *Averages Kill.* Proceedings of the 2001 Winter Simulation Conference, New Orleans.

6

The Role of Senior Leaders: Driving Sustainable Organizational Change

To improve is to change.
To be perfect is to change often.

Winston Churchill

The entire emergency department DMAIC team was so surprised that everyone looked in her direction when Joyce, the imaging director, declared that, in order to decrease patient blood order–to–blood draw time, her staff would draw blood before transferring emergency department patients. The DMAIC team leader asked, "You mean your techs have agreed to the additional task of drawing blood before they transport patients to imaging or roll in the portable?" Joyce replied, "Yes, they understand the importance of our team's mission, and we have already arranged for them to be trained in blood draws next week."

The 100-Day Workout process, as noted in Chapter 4, contains many safeguards to alert senior leaders when managers fall behind their committed action plans. One safeguard is for the senior leader to meet with managers who are behind within a week of the missed milestone. Franklin, a senior vice president at a midsized California facility, maintained his managers on schedule through the 100-Day Workout 30-day Check-in, but at the 60-day Check-in, he advised his managers that he would need to reschedule the support meeting for a week. The meeting was rescheduled to a time convenient to all. About an hour before the meeting, he advised his administrative assistant to reschedule the meeting in another three weeks. By the time of the 90-day Check-in, most of his managers were behind, some significantly so. He scheduled a supplemental meeting with his direct reports, in accordance with the 100-Day Workout protocol, but, again, it was canceled. The COO, who was the organization's leader of the 100-Day Workout process, allowed this behavior to continue throughout the next

100-Day Workout. The result was the organization fell short of its goal and significantly short of agreed-upon comparative benchmark. In an interview later, the CEO said something like, "The managers simply will not engage in the process. If they will not buy in, what can we do?"

Stories like these, which strike at both ends of the change acceptance process, are commonplace. Why does one group engage even radical change and another group fail?

Mistakes common to failed change initiatives have been well documented by Kotter and others over many years of research. Generally, Kotter (1996) puts failures into one or more of the following categories:

- Allowing too much complacency

- Failing to engage a broad-based management-staff guiding coalition to drive the change process

- Inadequately articulating vision for change urgency

- Undercommunicating the vision by a factor of 10

- Permitting obstacles to block the new vision

- Failing to create short-term wins

- Declaring victory too soon

- Neglecting to anchor changes firmly in the corporate culture

Cabana (1999) provides one of the most interesting glimpses into why physicians resist change. In the summation of his study, he affinitized reasons for lack of clinical guideline acceptance into three categories: lack of knowledge, attitudinal factors, and behavioral factors. Of note were the following citations:

- Lack of agreement with the aims overall change process

- Lack of agreement with a specific change

- Disbelief that the change will lead to desired results and/or adverse consequences

- Lack of motivating factors to support the change

Not all change is viewed negatively. In the three weeks before the 2005 Super Bowl, manufacturers were deluged with orders for high definition televisions, despite the fact that installation requires many hours of programming, significant changes to existing attachments, and relearning of operational requirements.

Some dieters, a minority to be sure, endure total life upheaval to attain their desired state.

So why is that some changes succeed and others fail?

When thought of in the context of TVs and diets, or physician acceptance and senior leader roles, the answer is fairly simple. As any good salesman might advise, successful change requires outweighing the costs of change—all the aggravation, uncertainty, and stress—with benefits received. So, how might we design a change system that seeks to outweigh costs over benefits in the context of a Lean–Six Sigma initiative?

Lewin (Caldwell 1996), in his Force Field process so common in quality method tool kits, breaks down the change process into three phases—Current State, Transition State, and Future State—making the case that the Transition State must involve building a strong case for change and the benefits for the desired Future State.

Kotter (1996) cites eight stages in his change process:

1. Making the case for change by establishing a sense of urgency, or the "burning platform" for change

2. Creating a guiding coalition of management and staff

3. Developing a vision

4. Communicating the vision and urgency of change to all levels and via multiple channels

5. Empowering employees to make independent change

6. Generating short-term wins

7. Consolidating gains and producing more change

8. Anchoring new approaches in the culture

Observing the factors leading to GE's radical transformation in the 1990s, Jacquie Vierling-Huang, GE's manager of workout, names four factors (Senge 1999, 82):

- They incorporated all staff into change initiatives. As Jack Welch said, "Get everyone in the game" (Caldwell 2005).

- They implemented best practices from inside and outside the company.

- They revised the staff evaluation process to include accomplishment of goals and behaviors supportive of the change.

- They set "stretch goals."

The *Good to Great in Healthcare* analysis (Caldwell 2004) found that those organizations achieving top-quartile performance had mastered three core processes:

- Behavioral attributes/role clarity

- Non-negotiable goal setting using aggressive comparative data

- Accountability systems

Kotter (2002, 1) notes that "people change what they do less because they are given analysis that shifts their *thinking* than because they are shown a truth that influences their *feelings*." This observation bears reflection. It is rarely analytical evidence that wins the day, although data is a vital step, but rather translating the case for change into meaningful benefits to those who must endure the steps to the desired state.

Consolidating the above thoughts into actionable categories leads us to the fact that effective change must involve two sets of activities. The first seeks to alter behaviors, but the strongest belief system is inadequate to drive sustainable change. We must also deploy change systems in the form of methods, tools, and infrastructure.

To optimize the power of Lean–Six Sigma, senior leaders are encouraged to adopt all or a major portion of the activities in the following two sections.

BEHAVIORAL ACTIVITIES

- Adopt a Tight-Loose-Tight change management philosophy as found in the *Good to Great in Healthcare* organizations (Caldwell 2004). Popularized by the Healthcare Advisory Board in the mid-1990s, Tight-Loose-Tight describes the process of successful change initiatives:

  - The first "Tight" refers to deployment of a non-negotiable goal-setting process, rigorously supported by aggressive comparative data and rapid cycle action planning.

  - The "Loose" refers to the decentralization to achieve the goal through actions and means.

  - The final "Tight" suggests accountability to achieve the non-negotiable goal in the time frame specified.

  - In other words, a senior leader might say, "Our first 'Tight' means that we have agreed on the comparative data analysis process and here are our non-negotiable goals. Each manager is empowered to implement whatever changes are appropriate to achieve their goal, which is our 'Loose.' However, while VPs and managers have the privilege of determining their own action plans, they are also accountable for hitting the target."

- Take steps to ensure that comparative data gaps of all types— organizationwide gaps such as productivity variances and patient satisfaction scores below goal and department-specific gaps such as lab charting time—are viewed as a call to action. Here we are seeking a culture that any performance variance demands action.

- As suggested by Kotter (1996), translate numerical goals into a strong case for change in terms of benefits received by the organization, by the manager, by the staff, and by the customers.

- Form an advisory team made up of managers and staff to implement an action plan to change key behaviors within the organization (as discussed in Chapter 1):

  – Status quo is never an option. Change is part of everyday work (versus protection of the status quo).

  – Time is of the essence; we simply cannot waste time when changing.

  – Role modification is often best for patient care (for example, imaging techs drawing blood in the ED).

  – Errors are unacceptable, and we must declare war on errors.

  – Care protocols here are always based on evidence-based medicine, and we insist on management by fact, not anecdote.

- Deploy effective multichannel communications to all stakeholder groups, and frequently and informally assess their effectiveness.

- Provide managers tools to conduct department visioning sessions aimed at achieving the desired behaviors described, using the Appreciative Inquiry approach (Hammond). The Appreciative Inquiry method engages staff to reflect upon a time when care was at its best, record the circumstances and factors that made "best" possible, and then build action plans to achieve these behavioral changes. (A two-hour agenda and facilitator guidelines for conducting an Appreciative Inquiry session appear on the CD.)

- Develop a standardized process that all senior leaders (executives, vice presidents, and directors) follow to support and coach managers who fall behind in their 100-Day Workout action plans or DMAIC implementation commitments.

CHANGE SYSTEMS

- Standardize project methods that share the characteristics of speed of implementation/"quick wins," accountability, and being driven by data, as suggested by Kotter (2002). The 100-Day Workout method, discussed in detail in Chapter 3, is an ideal method for achieving these aims.

- Establish a non-negotiable goal-setting process based on aggressive comparative data.

- Publicly post the results achieved.

- Reward and make "heroes" of those who exceed goals.

SUMMARY

Sustainable change has been an elusive accomplishment for many senior leaders for many years. Change research, in a search for replicable systems, has enjoyed less success. Many things that are difficult to achieve remain nonetheless vital, however, and change perhaps heads that list. The secret is never give up and never give in. Continue to experiment and try new approaches to generate enthusiasm for the change agenda, keeping those behavioral and structural factors that work and rejecting those that do not.

CHECKLISTS AND TOOLS ACCESSIBLE ELECTRONICALLY

- "Appreciative Inquiry Agenda and Facilitator Instructions"—on the CD

REFERENCES

Cabana, Michael. 1999. *JAMA*. 282(15): 1458–1465.

Caldwell, Chip. 1996. *Mentoring Strategic Change*. Milwaukee: ASQ Quality Press, 14,19.

————. 2004. "Good to Great in Healthcare: A Research Initiative." Conference presented by the American College of Healthcare Executives, St. Louis, May 26, 2004.

————. 2005. "Improving Throughput and Costs Using Lean–Six Sigma." Conference presented by the American College of Healthcare Executives, Phoenix, March 7–8, 2005.

Hammond, Sue A. 1996. *The Thin Book of Appreciative Inquiry*. Plano, TX: Thin Book Publishing.

Kotter, John P. 1996. *Leading Change*. Boston: Harvard Business School Press.

————. 2002. *The Heart of Change*. Boston: Harvard Business Press.

Pieper, Shannon. 2004. "Good to Great in Healthcare" *Healthcare Executive*. Chicago: Health Administration Press, 19(3): 21–26.

Senge, Peter. 1999. *The Dance of Change*. New York: Doubleday.

ADDITIONAL READING

Organization Influence Processes. Porter, L. W., Harold Angle, and Robert Allen. 2003. Armonk, NY: M. E. Sharp Publishers.

Good to Great. Collins, Jim. 2001. New York: HarperCollins.1995.

Danger in the Comfort Zone. Bardwick, Judith M. 1995. New York: AMACOM.

Organizational Change: Theory and Practice. Burke, W. Warner. 2002. Thousand Oaks, CA: Sage Publications.

The Tipping Point. Gladwell, Malcolm. 2002. New York: Back Bay Books.

The Thin Book of Appreciative Inquiry. Hammond, Sue A. 1996. Plano, TX: Thin Book Publishing.

The Servant as Leader. Greenleaf, Robert. 1991. Indianapolis: Robert Greenleaf Center.

Leadership: The Inner Side of Greatness. Koestenbaum, Peter. 1991. San Francisco: Jossey-Bass Publishing.

The Dance of Change. Senge, Peter. 1999. New York: Doubleday.

The Handbook for Managing Change in Healthcare. Caldwell, Chip. 1998. Milwaukee: ASQ Quality Press.

7

The Role of Senior Leaders: Engaging Physicians

If the people don't want to come out to the ballpark, nobody's going to stop them.

Yogi Berra

It goes without saying, but healthcare is one of the most complicated industries in which to build quality systems. Most Lean–Six Sigma Black Belts from outside healthcare fail because of this complexity, after having initially remarked that all industries are alike in that they all manage processes. While this is true, of course, these Black Belts quickly become frustrated because of the confusing role of physicians. In fact, in simply constructing a SIPOC diagram (supplier-inputs-processes-outputs-customer), attempting to place physicians in their proper roles can cause headaches. Only a handful of process changes can be fully optimized without physician engagement, and active management of the role of physicians may be one of the most vital tasks of senior leaders.

Case in Point 1: The emergency department at Morton Plant Medical Center in Clearwater, FL, faced an unreasonable number of patients leaving without treatment, leading to over $5 million in lost revenue and creating patient satisfaction scores just above the 60th percentile. Further, the relationships among ED nurses, inpatient unit nurses, ED physicians, and other caregivers were constantly under stress, at one point resulting in a finger-pointing session between ED nurses and ED physicians regarding who was to blame. Chartered by CEO Phil Beauchamp and Chief Nursing Executive Lisa Johnson, Dr. Brian Cook, the physician director, and Donna Moran, the nursing manager, formed a DMAIC team composed of four 100-Day Workout teams focusing on specific ED subprocesses. From the outset, Dr. Cook clearly established leadership, devoting significant time to review data with subteam leaders, coaching them in developing 100-Day Workout action plans, and overseeing rapid implementation of committed tasks. He resolved internal and external barriers to suggested process pilots by personally meeting with inpatient unit nurse managers, ancillary department directors, physician leaders, and other stakeholders to communicate the ED's goals and routes of collaboration by those in the care stream. Within a year, ED patient satisfaction topped the 90th percentile, a 50 percent gain; ED LOS dropped 25 percent; and Cost of Quality recovery exceeded $5 million. So, what did Dr. Cook, in concert with Donna, Lisa, and Phil, do to achieve the world-class improvements? He flawlessly executed the following roles:

- Restated the CEO/CNO vision into ED staff terms.

- Sought statistically valid process drivers around which to craft detailed 100-Day Workout action plans and appoint team leadership.

- Collaborated with internal and external leaders and stakeholders to set agreed-upon expectations.

- Created the infrastructure to create and track 100-Day Workout action plans.

- Resolved staff resistance to change, paradigm constraints, and delays.

- Led the celebration of achievements and shared praise with all involved.

Case in Point 2: A medical center in Mississippi discovered that improving care of patients with heart failure and shock (DRG 127) would recover over $1 million in Cost of Quality. Variation in medication utilization explained almost 90 percent of the variation in cost, as shown in Figure 7.1.

Further analysis demonstrated that, as shown in Figure 7.2, adequate variation in drug use warranted an attempt at uncovering sources of variation and engaging key stakeholders in aggressive action.

As pre-work, the DMAIC team analyzed medications used in great detail and discussed project success factors and risk factors. They concluded, as shown in Figure 7.3, that three critical roles would drive the success of reducing variation in medications use: physicians, case managers, and pharmacists. Although clinical pharmacists were actively involved in care processes, they had resisted being involved in clinical cost management activities, and case manager involvement had until this point focused on discharge management, not on clinical utilization. However, managers for pharmacy and case management felt that their staffs would engage if the physicians were engaged.

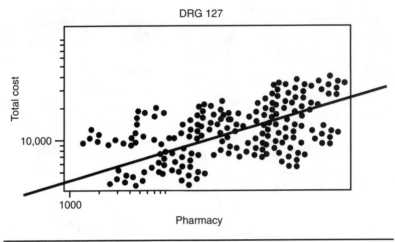

Figure 7.1   Scatter plot of total cost to pharmacy cost.

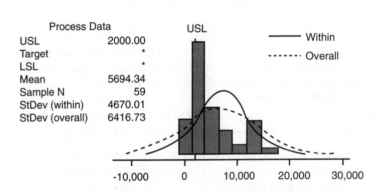

Figure 7.2   Drug cost distribution.

The chief medical officer agreed with the team that the leading admitter and informal physician leader would be the best at leading the DMAIC team. When he was approached, his general reaction was positive and he asked for examples of standing orders and protocols from other organizations with less variation. Several physicians were asked to attend an initial meeting. A second meeting produced a pilot standing order to be suggested to those physicians treating a high number of DRG 127 patients.

Level of commitment	Physician	Case manager	Pharmacist
Enthusiastic support	●	●	●
Help it work			
Agree		■	
Hesitant			
Indifferent	■		
Opposed			
Hostile			
Not currently involved			■

Figure 7.3   Stakeholder buy-in analysis.

After more than six meetings held over six months, almost no physicians, including the physicians authoring the standing order, used the protocol. The physician leader said that many improvements were more important than medication use in DRG 127 and that this project was unworthy of additional time and energy. The hospital recovered none of the more than $1 million opportunity.

Case in Point 3: A leading academic center in Florida determined that emergency department length-of-stay (LOS) improvement would yield over $5 million in reduced nurse worked hours per ED visit and reclaimed patients who were leaving before completing treatment (LWOT, or left without treatment). Based upon analysis of ED data, the physician and nurse managers charted a three-pronged approach to reduce ED LOS:

1. Reduce bottlenecks and delays in flow, particularly "time to ED bed" and "time from ED physician initial assessment to request for inpatient bed."

2. Reduce 50 percent of the variation in nurse staffing to hour-by-hour patient demand.

3. Reduce 50 percent of the variation in ED physician LOS variation.

The analysis of physician variation found significant unexplained differences in clinical practice (Figure 7.4).

However, at the initial meeting, a general apathy and resentment was apparent among most of the physicians. One of the more respected physicians said that it was unimportant how long the patient stayed and that she

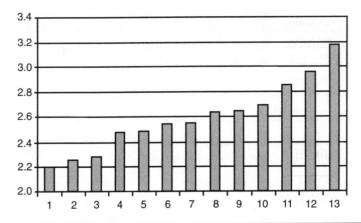

Figure 7.4 Emergency department physician LOS variation.

ordered a lot of tests unrelated to the patient's primary complaint because many patients did not have adequate primary care and she believed that quality care required her to order preventive tests. She went on to advise her colleagues that if the medical center prevented her from this primary physician role in conducting her ED physician episodic care duties, she might be forced to find work at a hospital that valued "quality" care. Despite this initial setback, a second meeting was planned, but the emergency physician rescheduled it at the last minute to be held 30 days later; a week before this meeting, he canceled it again.

Although physicians are indeed part of the healthcare system managed by the medical center, often this fact is not recognized. Some physicians even resist the notion that their actions affect other processes within the system, such as nursing, pharmacy, medical records, or billing and collections. Many are aware of the effect of their processes on medical center processes, but they prefer to ignore it. However, one important reason that physicians resist change is that the change frequently places more burdens on their processes—consuming more time, increasing complexity, providing less service to them or their patients. It is often the case that medical center leaders do not fully understand the physicians' processes before brainstorming potential changes. As a first step, leaders can go a long way toward averting resistance by simply developing what Deming called "profound knowledge" of physicians' processes in the DMAIC "analyze" step before entering the "improve" phase.

While the reasons for the reactions by these physicians varied significantly and were complex, the analysis revealed a lot about the physicians' role in organizationwide improvement efforts. By and large, disengagement by physicians can be attributed to a relatively few causes:

1. Not vested in the intended outcome (Cabana 1999).

2. Not understanding systems thinking or process analysis.

3. A bias that more resources and more staff are the best solutions and that analysis is a waste of time.

4. Adverse effect on physician processes by processes that aid hospital improvement.

5. A feeling that they should be compensated for their activities benefiting the hospital.

6. A feeling that the priority should be to improve processes that benefit their practices within the hospital before the hospital benefits from bottom-line improvements.

7. Little consensus among physicians regarding priority focus areas or their solutions.

8. A lack of "team" in physician behavior patterns, even if the individual practice is within the same medical group.

How can healthcare leaders tip the scale toward more effective collaboration and engagement?

The answer is not simple, but it has a simple form. The most effective approaches for engaging physicians seem to be to:

- Seek to fully understand physician needs in general and within the specific process to be changed during the pre-work, define, and improve phases of the DMAIC project and learn the degree of support required. A useful tool for analyzing physician and other key stakeholder current and required positions regarding the change is shown in Figure 7.3.

- Seek to build trust. This probably sounds simple, but physician–hospital executive trust has dramatically eroded over the past decade. The reasons for this lack of trust between the parties are complex, but they have a simple form. In the quest to recover lost margins, executive teams have, sometimes necessarily, flown in the face of physician interests and desires. As a result, the collaborative model has deteriorated to the level that, in many cases, relationships are combative.

- Educate physicians in all aspects of healthcare management, financial management, regulatory environment, and competitive pressures with an aim to establish a true visioning partnership about the future (not just cursory staff meeting advisories of days gone by) (Schwartz 2002).

- Seek win-win projects, at least initially. That is, find projects that, if achieved, will delight physicians, usually in the form of improving the efficiency in physician-hospital interfacing processes. For example, as we determined in Chapter 4, in surgery, a significant long-term Magic Moment goal assigned to the chief nurse executive would be to increase the ratio of "cut to close" hours per week and staffed hours per week. Statistical analysis usually suggests a focus on 7:30 A.M. surgery start times, decreased case turnaround times, and increased accuracy of physician preference card picking (thereby reducing interoperative delays.) DMAIC charters seeking to improve each of the processes can be written to support those matters most important to surgeons, that is, delays. Decreasing surgeon downtime, as a charter, will usually be wildly embraced by a critical mass of surgeons, with the exhaust of reduced Cost of Quality (in the form of decreased nurse staffing before and between cases).

- Negotiate a quid pro quo in which the organization provides a concession in some other area in exchange for physician agreement to embrace the desired change.

- Seek out physician influencers (referrers, physicians with high credibility) to lead the way, instead of having hospital managers and/or executives lead the change.

- Integrate improvement work casually into existing physician committee and task force structures, replacing those agenda items that are discussion-oriented, nonaction-producing topics and scheduling JCAHO topics bimonthly or quarterly instead of monthly (unless mandated) to free up time for action-oriented work and follow-up. The 100-Day Workout action plan format or a modification is ideally suited for action tracking.

- Consider incentives. (Although beware that incentives are often effective in the short term, but once offered become expected. Hence, the absence becomes a demotivator.)

- Seek nonphysician caregivers to execute the change or influence physicians to embrace the change. For example, since ambulation on the first postoperative day is a statistically significant driver for patients receiving hip replacement surgery (DRG 209), physical therapists can be engaged to call surgeons on the day of surgery soliciting a physical therapy order.

In summary, these approaches, while not unique, are indeed time consuming and less optimized in many healthcare organizations than is required to fully realize the power of Lean–Six Sigma. Heroic process innovation simply cannot be realized without physician engagement.

RECOMMENDED LEARNING SESSION

Learning Session for a One-Hour Senior Leader Meeting

One member of the executive team should serve as the recorder, capturing feedback on a flipchart.

1. Each executive takes 10 minutes to review the list of ways to approach physicians and record opportunities to engage physician leaders in a current initiative using one or more of the techniques listed (or innovation of a technique not listed).

2. Go around the room, discussing ideas generated by the executive group.

3. What, if anything, can be done to elevate physician engagement in one or more of the initiatives discussed?

4. Who should act upon the engagement ideas discussed? (The recorder or another accountable executive team member should be asked to capture this action plan.)

5. Set aside an hour every one to three months to review the action plan for progress.

REFERENCES

Cabana, Michael. 1999. *JAMA* 282(15): 1458–1465.

Rath and Strong. 2000. *Six Sigma Pocket Guide*. Lexington, MA: Rath & Strong, 10.

Schwartz, Richard W., and Kenneth H. Cohn. 2002. "The Necessity for Physician Involvement in Strategic Planning in Healthcare Organizations." *The American Journal of Surgery* 184: 269–278.

8

The Role of Senior Leaders: Achieving Sustainable Results (Magic Moment Example)

*The most difficult part of doing nothing
is not knowing when you're finished.*

Nelson DeMille, *Plum Island*

As observed earlier, one of the major missteps made by executive leaders in Lean-Six Sigma deployments is to behave as if Lean-Six Sigma is simply a project methodology. In many instances this is the fault of consultants who may be exceptional Black Belts but who have never served in a senior leadership capacity in healthcare and led executive teams down the path of selecting projects. This misstep is the kiss of death for any Lean-Six Sigma initiative. Executives may play this role for a few months, perhaps even a year, but sooner or later executives will begin to skip steering committee meetings, engage in side talk, or leave early. This occurs not because executives do not value their own contributions, but rather because executives begin to realize that project selection by committee is not a role that can remain top of mind for an effective executive. However, as Dr. Joseph Juran observed, "Results happen one project at a time and in no other way" (Caldwell 2004a). Therefore, to effectively maintain the Lean-Six Sigma infrastructure, executives need to have some sense of the potential impact of Lean-Six Sigma project methods. This chapter cites a case example that provides some sense of the structure, project activities, analysis issues, and results potential of a Lean-Six Sigma project.

MORTON PLANT HOSPITAL

Sitting at his desk, Phil Beauchamp, CEO of Morton Plant Hospital in Clearwater, FL, reviewed emergency department performance indicators with Lisa Johnson, vice president of patient services, and a Lean-Six Sigma consultant (Caldwell 2003b). While ED patient satisfaction was near the national average, at Morton Plant *average* is not in the management glossary. At that moment, Beauchamp committed himself and all the resources that might be required to help the ED leadership become world class.

Having won the prestigious Florida Sterling Quality Award and becoming the first U.S. hospital to be recognized in all categories of the Top 100 lists, the executive team and middle management at Morton Plant possess a passion to be recognized in their community and around the nation for providing high-quality care while minimizing waste due to poor quality. Adopting Lean-Six Sigma as a key deployment methodology to achieve its goal of becoming world class, Morton Plant took another step in its quality evolution.

Case Study Organization

Morton Plant Medical Center, Clearwater, FL

- 687-bed tertiary-care center, level II ED

- More than 50,000 ED visits annually

- First U.S. hospital to win all categories of Top 100

- Sterling Quality Award (Baldrige-based)

What They Accomplished

While still on the road to becoming world class, during the first year of deployment Morton Plant achieved these noteworthy results:

- Improved patient satisfaction more than 50%, from 61% to 95%

- Decreased length of stay 21% in the main ED and 61% in Express Care, the hospital's fast-track urgent care section of the ED

- Decreased left without treatment (LWOT) from 3.9% to below 0.5%, from a high of 212 to a new low of 7 per month

- Recovered more than $4 million in Cost of Quality through LWOT reduction alone

How Did They Get There?

The answer to the question of how Morton Plant achieved such outstanding results is not simple, but it has a simple form. Morton Plant became passionate about becoming a world-class hospital versus accepting the mediocrity symbolized by remaining at the average. This observation bears repetition. The hospital's managers decided that they wanted to be world class and that average was no longer a desired state. To achieve results, they:

- Established a three-year ED length-of-stay (LOS) stretch goal.

- Organized four Lean-Six Sigma teams, established team goals supporting the overall ED LOS three-year stretch goal, and established a project template enabling each team to select process changes that could be accomplished in the next 100 days (the 100-Day Workout approach).

- Changed the staff belief system from being "good enough" to one in which every key stakeholder was committed to achieving recognition as a world-class ED. A part of this activity was an "ER1" campaign in which physicians and staff, as well as key departments such as lab and imaging, participated in defining behaviors, roles, and measurements and in learning Lean-Six Sigma concepts necessary to achieve quantum improvement.

- Prioritized process improvement opportunities, using a Lean-Six Sigma analysis from a 14-day longitudinal study suggesting subprocesses that had a high statistical correlation to their overall strategic ED LOS goal.

- Selected a bite-sized subprocess goal for core process teams for each 100-Day period.

- Decided what *not* to focus on.

- Trained leaders and team members in Lean-Six Sigma engineering solution set development, project management, 100-Day Plan, and failure mode effects analysis (FMEA) and provided easy-to-use templates.

- Planned the deployment milestones for the entire 100-day period instead of simply setting up a biweekly meeting schedule.

Established a Three-year Stretch Goal

For long-term critical strategies, it is preferable that the CEO, but at a minimum a vice president who is accountable, becomes intimately involved in establishing the three-year stretch goal. Capitalizing on the power of Lean-Six Sigma thinking as a strategic tool, Beauchamp and Johnson recognized the ED as a critical entry point for admissions to Morton Plant and as a driver of the hospital's reputation in the community. Their designation of the ED as a "front door" to the organization distinguished the department as strategically important. Not every process in the organization can be included in the strategic short list.

Prioritization is necessary to keep management's attention from being diluted beyond reasonable control. This dilution factor was found to be a critical factor among underperformers in a *Good to Great in Healthcare* study of 220 healthcare organizations (Pieper 2004). Executives, even with good intentions, have the tendency to simply put too much on their collective plates, with the result being poor execution and follow-through. Consequently, they are unable to accomplish some of their critical goals. This pitfall can be avoided by identifying core business processes that yield high-leverage results for management efforts and focusing adequate time and attention on them. Core business processes in most hospitals include:

- Surgical services

- Diagnostics

- Emergency services

- Scheduling and registration

- Patient care throughput (length of stay and discharge time of day)

- Care management/clinical decision making

- Operations/supply chain

- Revenue cycle

- Intake services (physician offices, some outpatient functions, and others that feed into acute-care core processes)

A three-year strategic stretch goal can be determined for each of these core processes. Ownership of the goal must be assigned to an accountable vice president to deploy resources as needed to achieve the goal.

Examples of resources that Morton Plant used to progress toward its ED stretch goals include Lean-Six Sigma facilitation, information technology (IT) support, facility renovation, and leadership development efforts. Beyond supplying these resources, senior leaders relied on ED leadership and staff to fuel the improvement efforts.

Once the CEO and patient-care vice president prioritized ED, an intensive process of benchmarking began. EDs are among the easiest of core processes for which to obtain external, valid comparative data. Morton Plant used Healthcare Advisory Board research, Voluntary Hospitals of America (VHA) benchmarks, and comparable facilities known to them to determine its three-year stretch targets of length of stay, the key driver of patient satisfaction in EDs.

Using Lean-Six Sigma logic, Morton Plant came to recognize that setting a benchmark for average LOS was not a productive exercise. Setting goals around average performance is a bit like stating, "I have one foot in hot water and the other in ice water, but on average I feel pretty comfortable." Morton Plant applied this understanding and defined its goals in terms of the maximum acceptable LOS. In Lean-Six Sigma terminology, this quality threshold is referred to as the upper specification limit (USL), the point beyond which LOS should not exceed. What USL actually represents is the "voice of the customer." This approach especially appealed to senior leadership, who customarily would hear complaints from customers whose upper specification limit, or tolerance, had been exceeded. What better goal than to eliminate those outliers and horror stories of outrageous waits?

Based upon the external benchmarks, the three-year USL goal was set at 250 minutes, or just over four hours. In the Lean-Six Sigma strategy deployment approach, this means that the ED leadership was charged to redesign its critical subprocesses to ensure that 99.9997 percent of ED patients were treated within 250 minutes.

Organized Lean-Six Sigma Team Goals Around the Three-year Stretch Goal

Rather than follow the more common Lean-Six Sigma approach of completing one project and then deciding what to do next, Morton Plant laid its projects out in 100-day increments over a three-year period and reevaluated them at the end of each 100-day cycle. These projects, using the 100-Day Workout methodology, sought to execute quickly those changes that could have an effect within 100 days. Figure 8.1 illustrates this strategic approach.

The first challenge of Morton Plant's senior management was to ensure that effective leadership was on board within the ED. The best-selling management book *Good to Great* by Jim Collins (2001) lists this as one of the most vital factors present in organizations that achieve quantum improvement.

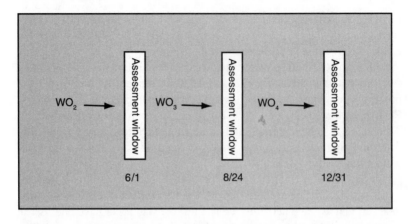

Figure 8.1 100-Day Workout annual plan.

Care was taken to avoid polarizing the interests of the hospital and the physician groups. ED medical director Brian Cook, MD, reported directly to the patient-care vice president, and compensation was designed to align incentives. Together, Cook and ED patient care director Donna Moran were given ownership of the stretch goal and charged with structuring the long-term approach to achieve the 250-minute USL.

The second task was to construct a high-level ED process flow, using the Lean-Six Sigma supplier-input-process-output-customer (SIPOC) tool. The result of this activity was a validation that four critical subprocesses must be synchronized and integrated to achieve the stretch goal. These processes were "patient entry to ED bed," "ED bed to diagnosis," "diagnosis to discharge," and "fast track." Obviously, these mirror the subprocesses selected by many well-publicized ED process improvement efforts (Healthcare Advisory Board 1999). Yet the exercise of displaying the process flow and selecting the critical subprocesses to measure was important in getting the teams' members to buy in. The critical-to-quality characteristic of "number of minutes to patient seen by physician" was discussed and validated with references.

The next step involved collecting adequate data on the Morton Plant ED's "current reality" to determine which processes influenced overall LOS the most. While the hospital's current data systems were valuable for patient flow, they provided only average LOS and cycle times and were inadequate for Lean-Six Sigma work. The need for data to drive change in the USL requires that Lean-Six Sigma staff or outside resources knowledgeable of Lean-Six Sigma concepts be engaged early in the process of IT system selection and design.

To overcome the weakness of available data, a 14-day longitudinal data collection was undertaken. Based on the 14-day study, a three-year goal was established for each of the subprocesses identified. This technique was invaluable in ensuring early success for the teams and also preventing frustrations from misguided efforts. Simply benchmarking other organizations to replicate their areas of focus can derail Lean-Six Sigma efforts. One benchmark organization that Morton Plant studied had made great strides by reducing x-ray cycle times. Had Morton Plant followed that path without first validating the relevance of x-ray to its overall stretch goal, substantial efforts would have been expended for a maximum potential improvement of only 14 minutes. The variation at Morton Plant from its fastest x-ray cycle time to its slowest was only 14 minutes. Hence, x-ray was not a logical focus at Morton Plant. Rather, the 14-day study found that "ED bed to test order," "CT cycle time," and "time to request an inpatient bed" were statistically among their top drivers. These became targets of the teams' action steps during successive 100-day cycles.

The next task was to establish the most effective infrastructure to achieve the stretch goals. As an oversight body, the Emergency Room Improvement Council (ERIC), accountable to the CEO and patient care VP, was established. Chaired by the ED medical director, the ERIC was charged to present its results every 100 days to the executive team and on occasion to the hospital's board of trustees. An internal leader with potential to drive radical improvement was appointed for each subprocess. Two leaders were physicians and two were charge nurses. These leaders were coached and became progressively more skilled at appointing representative staff to their teams and facilitating the teams in achieving 100-day action steps leading toward accomplishment of the three-year stretch goals.

The final task in this phase was the creation of a project management structure intended to maximize the productivity of the teams' efforts and to track performance. For their purposes, the 100-Day Workout was selected to lay out interim goals. Project activity is chartered in 100-day increments, with bite-sized and achievable milestones.

Changed the Staff Belief System

The belief system of the ED staff had to be changed from "good enough" performance to a world-class performance mind-set. Of all the activities, the belief system transformation effort was the most time-consuming, yet vital. The ED medical director, patient care director, charge nurses, and each team leader were oriented to Lean-Six Sigma flow analysis, improvement techniques, and implementation success factors contained within the 100-Day Workout method. Further, during a three-hour kickoff retreat and at many subsequent general staff meetings, each ED staff person and key staff members in lab and imaging were brought together to discuss the current and required belief systems and the behaviors that must exist for the world-class benchmarks to be achieved. The behaviors identified during this kickoff session were measured for a baseline and periodically over the next two years.

Prioritized Process Improvement Opportunities

Morton Plant prioritized its process improvement opportunities based on the Lean-Six Sigma analysis template instead of the less rigorous PDCA approach or the approach of copying best practices found in the literature or provided by national benchmarking organizations. Traditional improvement approaches involve less rigorous design of experiments (DOE) techniques than typically are used in Lean-Six Sigma projects. The hierarchy of DOE techniques, in ascending order of sophistication, is as follows:

- *"Shoot from the Hip"*—While this is not actually a recognized DOE technique, process change without any data to support the change concept is the most commonly observed. This "let's just do something" mentality seems to exist among physician teams as well as operations teams. It is as if physicians, once they leave the patient care areas, often abandon their scientific approach to clinical problem solving. No physician would treat a patient's pathophysiology without rigorous follow-up diagnostics to ensure the therapeutic regimen was effective. Yet, inside an improvement meeting, teams sometimes throw all scientific logic out the window, searching for the first quick fix.

- *Trial and Error of Best Practices*—Using improvement practices found in the literature, at meetings, or through benchmarking services like the Healthcare Advisory Board can provide a rich solution set for a team to brainstorm. However, application of these best practices without first understanding the major sources of variation within an organization's own processes can lead to wasted effort.

- *Simple Regression Analysis*—In what the Lean-Six Sigma project methodology refers to as critical-to-quality (CTQ) characteristics, an effort is made to uncover those subprocesses that, if improved, will likely lead to improvement of overall process performance. For example, at Morton Plant it was discovered that if all tests could be ordered within 45 minutes, there was a significant probability that the total LOS would not exceed 250 minutes.

- *Multivariate Regression Analysis*—Similar to simple regression, multivariate regression analysis examines combinations of factors.

- *Rapid Cycle Experiments*—Using two sample t-tests or simply run charting of only 25 data points (Langley 1996, 110), teams can evaluate multiple process change concepts sequentially by sampling just a few tests of change per day or shift to determine the optimum mix of change ideas.

- *Lean Six Sigma Simulation*—Not often considered by statisticians to be part of the DOE suite, simulation allows for the testing of potential improvements without actually going through the sometimes traumatic process of piloting. While expensive and conducted best by experienced statisticians and simulationists, simulation is particularly useful when throughput and staffing/capacity optimization are key.

Selected Bite-Sized Subprocess Goal for Each 100-Day Workout

Core process teams selected a bite-sized subprocess goal for each 100-Day Workout instead of trying to solve every opportunity presented by the data at once. For example, rather than trying to implement every item, the Admit Team set as one 100-Day Workout goal to implement—and implement flawlessly—a new form to request inpatient beds 80 minutes sooner in the patient stay.

Decided What Not to Focus On

The teams in the Morton Plant ED decided what *not* to focus on in their improvement efforts. This *Good to Great in Healthcare* factor was determined to be a vital one during research into quantum improvers versus non-starters (Pieper 2004). A common characteristic of nonstarter organizations is constantly planning and replanning, delaying implementation month by month until little or nothing is achieved.

Trained Leaders and Team Members

Morton Plant trained leaders and team members in Lean-Six Sigma engineering solution set development, project management, 100-Day Workout approach, and failure mode effects analysis (FMEA) and provided easy-to-use templates.

Planned Deployment Milestones

The teams at Morton Plant planned the deployment milestones for the entire 100-day period instead of setting up a biweekly meeting schedule with no predetermined purpose for each meeting. Again, *Good to Great in Healthcare* organizations are flawless planners; nonstarters are endless "meeters" (Pieper 2004). The Morton Plant teams began with the end in mind—their 100-Day Workout goal—and worked backward, ensuring that each critical milestone was determined and achieved.

The strategic deployment of Lean-Six Sigma, using a combination of project methods, primarily DMAIC and 100-Day Workout, enabled Morton Plant to improve patient satisfaction over 50%, reduce ED LOS by 21%, and recover over $4 million in Cost of Quality.

REFERENCES

Caldwell, Chip, and James Brexler. 2004. "Improving Throughput and Costs Using Lean-Six Sigma." Conference presented by the American College of Healthcare Executives, Key West, FL, January 12–13, 2004.

Caldwell, Chip, Lisa Johnson, Brian Cook, and Donna Moran. 2003. "ER Six Sigma Effort Results in 50% Satisfaction Improvement and $4 million Cost Recovery" [Online article; accessed June 6, 2004.] On CD, "Healthleaders Morton Plant ED Case Study."

Collins, Jim. 2001. *Good to Great.* New York: HarperCollins.

Healthcare Advisory Board. 1999. *The Clockwork ED.* Washington: Advisory Board Company.

Langley, Gerald, Kevin Nolan, Thomas Nolan, Clifford Norman, and Lloyd Provost. 1996. *The Improvement Guide.* San Francisco: Jossey-Bass Publishers.

Pieper, Shannon. 2004. "Good to Great in Healthcare." *Healthcare Executive* 19(3): 21–26.

ADDITIONAL READING

Quality Improvement Through Planned Experimentation. Moen, Ronald, Thomas Nolan, and Lloyd Provost. 1999. New York: McGraw Hill Professional Publishing.

The Improvement Guide. Langley, Gerald, Kevin Nolan, Thomas Nolan, Clifford Norman, and Lloyd Provost. 1996. San Francisco: Jossey-Bass Publishers, 106–112.

9
Summation

Never underestimate the magnitude of the
forces that reinforce the status quo.

John Kotter

A lot of ground has been covered in this book, and it is doubtful that a quick read or even a one-time thoughtful study will produce the requisite level of expertise to use all key aspects of the structured systems presented. However, the major tenets have a simple form.

To achieve success in the strategic deployment of Lean-Six Sigma—indeed, of any quality system—the serious senior leader or leadership team will begin with a few major tenets, as follows:

- Achieving maximum benefit of the power of Lean-Six Sigma is to recognize that, as an organizationwide commitment to achieve sustainable strategic results, the ownership of Lean-Six Sigma is a nondelegable role of senior leaders, with one executive named the accountable manager.

- A major first step is an assessment of the organization's current quality system(s) effectiveness and precise articulation of its strengths, weaknesses, and next level of growth.

- The importance of understanding the relationship between quality, throughput, and Cost of Quality and of training managers at all levels to recognize and root out waste in all its forms cannot be overstated.

- Translating resource goals into Magic Moment process goals is the only quality-based approach that focuses on the waste in processes.

In short, there is a time to assess the current and potential impact of Lean-Six Sigma on the organization's key priorities. Now is that time.

Glossary

The glossary is available in electronic format on the accompanying CD.

100-Day Workout—A highly effective type of project designed to implement all or part of a known process solution set within 100 days. A hallmark of the 100-Day Workout is the creation of an action plan during the 1 to 3 day kickoff that includes action items in categories of DO NOW, 30-day, 60-day, and 90-day.

Balanced Scorecard—The measurement tool used by the CEO Steering Council and core process accountable executives, along with the Magic Moment and Strategy Deployment Plans, to assess degree of accomplishment of strategic results and the effectiveness of projects.

Black Belt—A skilled individual charged to facilitate and provide sophisticated statistical and engineering analysis and solution sets. An individual earns a Black Belt designation through demonstrated accomplishment of project results using the DMAIC methodology and after having defended her/his successful Black Belt project to a Master Black Belt and passed a rigorous written examination.

Champion—An executive role accountable for a 3-year Magic Moment goal (see definition). It is the Champion's responsibility to lay out the project schedule aimed at achieving the Magic Moment strategic goal and to support the project leader and Green Belt or Black Belt in the completion of individual projects.

change concept—A set of generalized process redesign techniques that can be applied to achieve the aim (for example, match staffing to demand, shape demand, standardize, consolidate).

core process—One of ten to fifteen strategic care or business processes chosen to achieve long-term strategic results. A core process must be large enough to contain significant cost of quality and cost of poor quality with capacity to effectively conduct at least one DMAIC, one PDCA, and two Workouts simultaneously, yet small enough to be manageable. The long-term strategic goals for each core process is assigned to an accountable executive—this executive must oversee the conduct of a sufficient number of projects to achieve the six-month goal or charter additional activity to make up the gap. Examples of typical core processes are patient care throughput, revenue cycle, supply chain, evidence-based medical/clinical utilization, and management system/ staffing to demand.

Cost of Quality (COQ)—The cost incurred in a process to assure that the quality standard is met. These costs do not add value to the customer of the process but assure that high quality is achieved. Types of COQ include inspection and prevention costs. COQ should be kept as low as possible while maintaining a high level of quality. For example, if the quality standard is to deliver first dose antibiotics in 2 hours (plus or minus 10 minutes), then the process to deliver the antibiotic costs a certain amount, say $1000 per dose—including staff time, equipment, and the drug. The process also includes steps to assure that the antibiotic is delivered within 2 hours; these may include inspection steps by various staff, which might cost an additional $140 per dose. So the total cost of the process is $1140, including $140 in COQ costs.

Cost of Poor Quality (COPQ)—The cost incurred when processes fail. These costs include the cost of repeating the process to get it right; costs to explain what happened and how you will correct the problem to the patient, MD, and family; excessive malpractice costs; complaint management; risk management; legal costs; and so on. These costs are categorized as internal failures and external failures. In healthcare, the COPQ and COQ cost 33% of the typical budget. For example, if the goal is to deliver first dose antibiotics within 2 hours (plus or minus 10 minutes), some percentage will fail to meet the goal. The industry average is about 20% failure. Some process failures will cost more than others, but the cost of correcting an incorrect dose, route, patient, or drug will require another administration at a minimum, which costs $1140. If half require a second administration with a 20% failure rate, 10% of antibiotic administrations will be repeated (an additional $114 per dose). The total cost, including the process cost, COQ cost, and COPQ cost is $1254. Therefore, in this example, total COQ/COQP cost is 25.4% of the process cost. The aim is to reduce this cost as much as possible.

critical-to-quality (CTQ)—A process-specific measurable and measured process output/outcome that represents the "voice of the customer." The CTQ is statistically analyzed to determine those subprocesses that drive the CTQ (referred to as the key process input variable or KPIV).

Some Lean-Six Sigma textbooks refer to CTQ as the key process output variable (KPOV).

design of experiments (DOE)—A Lean-Six Sigma Black Belt tool to test the effectiveness of a process change upon a process output. For example, an ED might be curious if adding a specific lower extremity injury advance protocol to be executed by the triage nurse will decrease ED LOS for these diagnoses. After orienting the pilot triage nurse, the effectiveness of this change can be analyzed statistically over the next 25 lower extremity patients. It is generally best to test effectiveness of process change ideas in rapid cycle fashion—one shift, one day, three days—and not over an extended period of time. (Black Belts are schooled in sampling theory to ensure that effective hypotheses are not incorrectly rejected and that ineffective hypotheses are not incorrectly accepted.)

DMAIC—A Six Sigma improvement methodology. D-Define, M-Measure, A-Analyze, I-Improve, C-Control. The hallmarks of this workhorse Six Sigma methodology are statistical methods and a strong execution bias. Its weaknesses are a lack of strong flow engineering techniques, overcome through the introduction of the eight lean flow and capacity optimization solutions and highly variable change acceleration effectiveness, overcome through the introduction of Six Sigma design of experiments (DOE) simulation techniques.

DPMO—Defects per million opportunities, a measure used by manufacturing Black Belts to measure quality yields. This traditional metric has been utilized by manufacturing to measure quality many years before Six Sigma. It is simply how they measure quality. Unfortunately, unlike manufacturing, healthcare has no traditional quality measures based on "per million" anything. We simply do not produce a million medications or a million cardiac surgeries. Healthcare measures quality almost universally as a percentage (nosocomial infection rate, mortality rate, x-ray retake rate, overtime rate). In healthcare, the DPMO concept confuses nurses, physicians, and other staff and adds no value to the measurement of quality. Rather, it is best to convert the DPMO concept to a "per hundred" or percentage, which is easily understood by physicians, nurses, and others. DPMO is simply "per million" with 6 zeros; a percentage can be derived by moving the decimal four places to the left. For example, 3-sigma is 66,000 DPMO; to convert to a percentage, simply move the decimal four places to the left to produce 6.6%. All staff members understand 6.6%; none understand 66,000 DPMO.

key process input variable (KPIV)—The statistically determined subprocess predictor of a process CTQ metric (critical-to-quality) and is sometimes referred to as Critical 'x,' reflecting its critical impact on a CTQ.

The KPIV is usually reflected via a correlation analysis. For example, if our CTQ is for inpatients to be discharged no later than 2 PM, a KPIV would be a physician discharge order no later than 10 AM and another would be transportation arranged no later than 48 hours prior to expected discharge.

lean—A quality improvement concept designed to reduce waste and process cycle time. Lean rules include focusing on the customer "aim," avoiding batching if customers will be delayed, waste elimination, and continuous flow or "pull." Lean is generally not as effective as a stand-alone approach, but rather incorporated into Six Sigma, due to Six Sigma's more robust execution method, DMAIC.

lower specification limit (LSL)—A Lean-Six Sigma Black Belt and engineering designation for the "voice of the customer." For example, hand-washing below an LSL of 30 seconds dramatically decreases hand-washing effectiveness (based on CDC Guidelines), or time with physician less than 10 minutes yields patient complaints, or providing the patient noon meal no earlier than 11:30 AM yields patient complaints. The LSL travels with a companion, USL (upper specification limit). It is important to note that the LSL and USL are unrelated to the "voice of the process," or the ability of the process to predictably achieve customer requirements as measured by the LSL/USL. In other words, while the patient may want to be treated in the ED in no greater than four hours, an ED only capable of treating patients in five hours. This later "voice of the process" is signified by the Lean-Six Sigma Black Belt/engineering terminology lower capability limit (LCL) or upper capability limit (UCL).

Magic Moment—That strategic point in time, usually two to three years, against which all project results, effective use of technology, and other strategic and tactical plans produce a defined, focused, measurable result. Once the measures for the Magic Moment are confirmed and the critical 10 to 15 strategic core processes are determined and assigned to an accountable executive, milestone results are established in six-month increments, called waves. During each wave, executives oversee the completion of multiple projects within their core processes to reach the milestone goals. If, for any reason, projects slip or fail to achieve their targets summing up to the milestone results, executives must make up the difference in a process known as a Supplemental Workout.

non value added (NVA) cost—See **COPQ**.

PDCA—Plan, Do, Check, Act cycle of improvement created by Walter Shewart in the 1930s and enhanced by quality leaders like W. Edwards Deming and Joseph Juran over the years. Some organizations use Deming's version: PDSA, or Plan, Do, Study, Act. The impact of effective use of PDCA concepts in an organization is that the culture evolves to one of high creativity, experimentation, and defeat of the status quo.

project—A chartered activity intended to achieve a stated result aligned to a Magic Moment goal.

project charter—A statement of the purpose or expected result of the team's or manager's project during the fiscal year or that specific 100-day implementation period. An effective aim statement follows the SMART format (S = specific, including the process boundaries; M = measurable and measured; A = agreed upon by the manager and his/her supervisor; R = Realistic, yet stretch; T = time-specific, results to be achieved by a defined date).

quality formula—Once the quality standard is defined and the process created to achieve the quality standard, the equation for quality becomes process (work) divided by resource consumption. The goal of quality projects is to decrease the work and the resource in the same proportion so that "as quality goes up, costs go down." For example, if a respiratory therapy manager improves a treatment and saves 15 minutes per treatment in an organization that performs 25,000 treatments, then he saved 6250 hours of process work time. But with this change, the quality equation is out of balance by 6250 hours until either 2.2 FTEs are reduced or an additional 6250 hours of additional work is brought into the department. A similar example can be drawn from the relationship between medical error reduction and cost improvement.

quality yield—Percent quality standard achieved. Quality yield should be broadened to include productivity as well as process quality. For example, calculating the daily quality yield of staffing of variably staffed departments, based upon a quality-based staffing matrix, will illustrate that departments achieve their own definition of quality less than 50% of the time. Quality yields can be calculated on percentage of time ED achieves 3 hour LOS, percentage of time surgery achieves 7:30 AM start times or 15-minute turnover times, or the percentage of patient care/care management/discharge planning that achieve noon discharge. Each of these process variables, if improved, will produce cost of quality recovery as exhaust, thereby driving 100-Day Workout focus areas.

sigma quality levels—The common metric used by Black Belts to measure variation from the quality goal (LSL and USL). Example quality goals might be ED LOS less than four hours, 7:30 AM surgery start time, noon discharge, billing in less than five days (with no errors). Sigma levels can easily be converted to quality yield for ease of explanation. For example, 1-Sigma equals 33%, 1.5-Sigma equals 50%, 2-Sigma equals 69%, 3-Sigma equals 93%, and 6-Sigma equals 99.9997%.

SIPOC—A tabular form used by Black Belts to aid the team in understanding Suppliers-Inputs-Processes-Outputs-Customer. SIPOC is created in the "D"-Define step, but used frequently throughout the DMAIC project to clarify data collection, analysis, improvement ideas, and/or to keep the team focused on its goal(s).

SMART—S = specific, including the process boundaries; M = measurable and measured; A = agreed upon by the manager and his/her supervisor; R = realistic, yet stretch; T = time specific, results to be achieved by a defined date.

Supplemental 100-Day Workout—Highly focused 100-Day Workout launched in the event the quality and/or cost recovery goals are not achieved during a specific six-month wave. The go/no-go decision rests with the Champion.

upper specification limit (USL)—A Lean-Six Sigma Black Belt and engineering designation for the "voice of the customer." For example, treating an ED patient in less than four hours or providing the noon patient meal no later than 12:30 PM. The USL travels with a companion, LSL (lower specification limit). It is important to note that the LSL and USL are unrelated to the "voice of the process," or the ability of the process to predictably achieve customer requirements as measured by the LSL/USL. In other words, while the patient may desire to be treated in the ED in no greater than four hours, an ED capable of treating patients in five hours fails to meet customer needs. This later "voice of the process" is signified by the Lean-Six Sigma Black Belt/engineering terminology lower capability limit (LCL) or upper capability limit (UCL).

wave—A 100-day to six-month implementation window during which the Champion for each strategic core process launches DMAIC, PDCA, and/or multiple Workouts to achieve the strategic quality and cost recovery goals for that wave.

REFERENCES

Breyfogle, Forrest. 2003. *Implementing Six Sigma,* 2nd edition. Hoboken, NJ: John Wiley & Sons.

Caldwell, Chip, and James Brexler. 2004. "Improving Throughput and Costs Using Lean-Six Sigma." Conference presented for American College of Healthcare Executives, Key West, FL, January 12-13, 2004.

Langley, Gerald, Kevin Nolan, Thomas Nolan, Clifford Norman, and Lloyd Provost. 1996. *The Improvement Guide.* San Franciso: Jossey-Bass Publishers.

Pande, Peter, Robert Neuman, and Roland Cavanagh. 2000. *The Six Sigma Way.* New York: McGraw Hill.

Appendix A

Waste Walk Form

This form is used by a Black Belt or other facilitator to kick off an Operations Waste 100-Day Workout to stimulate changes that managers might implement to extract Cost of Quality (COQ).

An electronic version can be found on the CD.

Key point	Observations	Ideas to eliminate	Estimated cost recovered if eliminated
Overproduction/overcapacity (below stated goal level) **Staffing-to-demand** (greater than stated staffing ratio at this moment)			
Correction (inspection and rework)			
Processing			
Inventory			
Waiting			
Motion of people			
Material and information movement			

100-DAY WASTE WALK:
LEAN-SIX SIGMA CONCEPT WORKSHEET

(Excerpt of productivity improvement oriented change concepts from the Lean-Six Sigma Solution Set in Appendix C.)

Key point	Potential application	Estimated cost recovery if implemented	Who must approve?
1. Eliminate things that are not used			
2. Consolidate functions, job classifications			
3. Standardize (create a formal process)			
4. Eliminate multiple entry			
5. Reduce or eliminate overkill			
6. Recycle or reuse			
7. Use substitution			
8. Use constraints and forcing functions			
9. Use reminders			
10. Reduce classifications			
11. Apply default mode (only 1 way)			
12. Minimize handoffs.			
13. Adjust to peak and trough demand			
14. Reduce setup or startup time			
15. Move steps in the process close together			
16. Find and remove bottlenecks			
17. Match staffing to demand			
18. Shape demand			

Appendix B

DMAIC Project Charter Template

Date: _____

Project resources	Planned project milestone dates		Actual project milestone dates
Project champion James Barfeld, CNO **Process owner(s)** Marley Jones, ED director **Black Belt:** Lynne Sisak, MBB Brian Drake, GB	**Completed project charter:**	8/15	7/13
	Define:	8/15	7/24
	Measure:	9/15	8/24
	Analyze:	9/15	9/14
	Improve:	9/15–12/14	10/1
	Control:	12/31	12/30
DMAIC project overview			
Current state process performance validation	• ED LOS: GHC fm 2.6 to 2.24 KHC 3.2 to 2.7 • Productive hours /visit: GHC 2.09 to 1.9 KHC 2.5 to 2.08 • Cost per ED visit		
Opportunity/ problem statement *SMART format*	On both campuses, reduce 50% LOS gap above the median, reduce EDP LOS variation by 50%, reduce nurse staffing to demand by 50%, and reduce nurse FTEs by 5.2 (~ $380K) (14.9 hrs/day on each campus) as LOS drops 14% and 17%, respectively, by 12.14.		
Project scope *(Ensure project is not too large)* **Items in scope:** **Items out of scope:**	ED operations, including aligned Dx/Rx functions and inpatient bed assignment as well as staffing processes and staffing plans. Inpatient unit flow except for the bed assignment process.		

Continued

Desired process performance/goal of the improvement effort including cost recovery	• ED LOS: GHC fm 2.6 to 2.24 KHC 3.2 to 2.7 • Productive hours /visit: GHC 2.09 to 1.9 KHC 2.5 to 2.08
Business case analysis	
Reasons for doing this project now. Are there consequences of not doing this project now?	LOS varies significantly enough on both campuses to warrant a DMAIC project.

Current and potential key process indicators
Baseline measure
	1. ED patient flow
	  • Triage to EDP assess < 30 min (Marley J)
	  • 1st blood order–Result < 60 min (Rick A)
	  • 1st x-ray order–Result < 45 min (Zane K)
	  • Discharge orders–Discharge < 30 min (Marley J)
	  • EDP assess–Request for bed < 30m (Beals R)
	2. EDP LOS variation decr 50% (B. Rusk, MD)
	3. Nurse staffing: Worked Hours per ED visit (Marley J)
	  • Staffing to demand improve 50%
	  • Adjust RN staffing as LOS decreases by 14% at GCH and 17% at KHC, recovering 14.9 RN hours per day at each campus, totaling $380,020.

Business case analysis	
The key success factors for this project/expected benefits *Target savings, target metric reduction*	• **Productive hours /visit: GHC 2.09 to 1.9 KHC 2.5 to 2.08** • Adjust RN staffing as LOS decreases by 14% at GCH & 17% at KHC, recovering 5.6 FTEs (14.9 RN hours/day at each campus) totaling $380,020.
Hypothesized cost recovery/COPQ	5.6 FTEs, or 29.8 RN hours/day (14.9 at each campus), producing $380,020 Cost of Quality recovery.
Describe the strategic alignment of this project	Aligns with the vision to recover Cost of Quality to enable a new facility.
DMAIC project detail	
Stakeholders	ED physicians ED nurses and other clinical and administrative staff Lab personnel X-ray personnel Radiologists Bed control staff Inpatient unit nurse managers and nurses

Continued

Continued

Resources/team members and functional area	Marley J Beals R Zane K Rick A Nurse supervisors
Anticipated resources *Any staff, consultants, capital or associated costs*	No resources required other than one Black Belt and stakeholder availability
Deliverables to exec team *Driven by project plan and reported by process owner*	• **Productive hours /visit: GHC 2.09 to 1.9 KHC 2.5 to 2.08** • Adjust RN staffing as LOS decreases by 14% at GCH and 17% at KHC, recovering 14.9 hours/day at each campus, totaling $380,020.
Constraints *Possible limitations that will affect project outcomes*	• Lack of commitment/buy-in among key stakeholders; a "we could never try that here!" posture. • Time constraints due to JCAHO, others
Communication strategy *What will be communicated to whom (audience) and how (tactics)*	• ED physician monthly data update • Participating dept monthly meeting
Project charter change **Brief description of change**	*Revision #* *Date:*

Signatures of accountability *Dated signatures indicate agreement with the project charter content and shared accountability in meeting the project goals and timelines*	**Process owner** *Marley Jones*	**Black Belt** *Lynne Sisak*	**VP champion** *James Barfeld*	**COO** *Darlene Rooney*

Appendix C

Lean-Six Sigma Solution Set

Change Concepts optimize patient care throughput, reduce process lead times, trim dependent process cycle times and wait times, and, when combined with the Match Staffing to Demand Solution Set, recapture lost productivity and cost.

Process design techniques that optimize throughput and reduce lead time tend to focus on the following eight key strategies. They have the effect (shown by the directional arrows in the process map) of reducing dependent subprocess cycle time, initiating dependent subprocesses earlier in the core process, and/or parallel processing independent subprocesses.

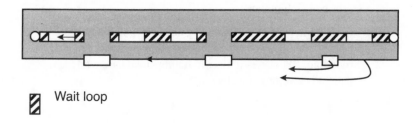

Wait loop

The eight strategies are:

1. Develop contingency plans for failure modes.

2. Consolidate functions/processes; eliminate steps.

3. Initiate dependent subprocesses earlier in the process.

4. Parallel process nondependent subprocesses.

5. Decrease subprocess cycle times.

6. Eliminate waste, errors, waits, and delays.

7. Match staffing and capacity to demand.

8. Shape demand.

DEVELOP CONTINGENCY PLANS
FOR FAILURE MODES

1. Determine critical processes, define failure criteria (for example, ED patients must have all diagnostic tests ordered within 45 minutes of their stay, and case managers must initiate discharge plans 24 hours *prior to* admission), and deploy "sensors" to know when failure modes hit.

   – Prepare backup or contingency plans to deal with unexpected delays.

   – Prepare a contingency plan for when a physician is called to ED or OR.

   – Failure mode that ED will transfer the patient to the assigned inpatient bed within 30 minutes of notification of bed assignment.

2. Cross-train staff to meet shifting demand (phlebotomists pass by pharmacy to carry stat meds to patient units while rounding; ED nurses initiate initial inpatient care while patient is awaiting transfer).

CONSOLIDATE FUNCTIONS/PROCESSES;
ELIMINATE STEPS

3. Consolidate or eliminate positions.

4. Reduce task, function, and inventory classifications.

5. Decrease job classifications/job types.

6. Use resources for more than one purpose. thereby eliminating a resource.

7. Reduce layers of supervision; increase span of control.

8. Eliminate multiple entry (instead of 22 access points to register, decrease to 5).

9. Reduce the number of components.

10. Minimize handoffs. (Change to "universal" bed versus critical care to acute care handoff. Eighty-one percent of medication errors occur at handoffs in care.)

11. Consider people to be in the same system. (Rather than let ED "complain" about delayed labs, x-ray, and CT, form a team to review the ED patient's total lapse time from entry through triage, first orders, test completion/results, and disposition orders to ultimate discharge/transfer from unit; provide registration leadership with total lapsed time analysis to include their processes and care processes.)

12. Use substitution.

13. Sort product into grades or classes.

14. Standardize.

INITIATE DEPENDENT SUBPROCESSES EARLIER

15. Work with suppliers.

16. Move decisions earlier in the process.

    – Give ED physician admitting authority, ability to initiate request for inpatient bed (HCAB 1999).

    – Give triage nurse authority to "pend" inpatient beds if preestablished criteria are met.

    – Create an ED preemptive bed request process (HCAB 1999).

    – Assign admitted patient from ED triage to hospitalist/admitting physician versus waiting until full ED workup is complete.

    – In ED, initiate the request for bed process no later than 30 minutes for ED physician initial exam (initiating the bed request process does not require the attending's visit or initial orders).

PARALLEL PROCESS NONDEPENDENT SUBPROCESSES

Examine processes to potentially perform a sequential subprocess in parallel with another process.

17. Parallel process nondependent subprocesses.

   – Prepare surgery suite for surgery while setting up instruments.

   – Obtain patient information during waiting times.

   – Begin discharge teaching during the admit process.

   – In ED, register patient at the bedside so that treatment processes can be initiated simultaneously (HCAB 1999).

   – In ED, use preemptive order guidelines (HCAB 1999).

18. Work with internal and external suppliers to synchronize delivery to point of need at time of need.

   – For ED admitted patients, begin the request for inpatient bed as soon as the ED physician recognizes the need for admission (versus waiting until all tests are returned and/or the admitting physician writes orders). The request for bed process is not dependent upon admitting physician orders.

DECREASE SUBPROCESS CYCLE TIME

19. Remove intermediaries.

20. Change target or set points. (In ED, launch a "10 minutes to world-class care" initiative, driving all key process owners to create breakthrough thinking to achieve no greater than 10 minutes to the next care step. In lab, lab manager will measure not just time after the specimen hits the lab, but rather time from physician order until results reviewed by physician.)

21. Move steps in the process close together.

   – Move radiography equipment next to the units and ED with high demand.

   – Move outpatient surgery (OPS) support to OPS area.

   – Move patient's chart to bedside.

– Examine the workflow of processes and relocate needed materials so that they are in the path of the process versus randomly placed in the room.

22. Find and remove bottlenecks.

23. Use automation.

– A "ready" inpatient bed automatically interfaces with the bed control system when the housekeeper dials into the phone system that the room is clean for the next patient, instead of waiting until the RN notifies admitting that the bed is ready.

– Use comparative data to determine potential opportunity areas.

– Use standard analysis software to determine staffing by shift, by day, and by season.

– Use standard software to schedule staff.

– Use handheld computers in preop testing.

– Deploy medication management bedside devices to eliminate manual MARs and unnecessary calls to physicians and pharmacy.

24. Smooth out the workflow.

– For ED admissions, redesign the admitting process to bypass bed control (HCAB 1999).

– In ED, use a triage short form versus a full workup to get the patient to the ED bed in five minutes (HCAB 1999).

– Implement a no-delay ED nurse report for ED inpatient transfers through a phone-based, recorded nurse report (HCAB 1999).

25. Extend specialist's time.

– Use the skills and expertise of each member of the primary care team. For example, receptionists are trained to schedule patients automatically for the appropriate type of appointment, rather than handing them off to the nurse.

– Use video and information technology to extend specialists' time.

- In ED, deploy a charting scribe to free up ED physician time and expedite workflow (HCAB 1999).

- Sort products into grades or classes.

ELIMINATE WASTE, ERRORS, WAITS, AND DELAYS

26. Eliminate things that are not used.

27. Eliminate multiple entry.

28. Reduce or eliminate overkill.

29. Recycle or reuse.

30. Use substitution.

31. Listen to customers.

32. Focus on the outcome to a customer.

33. Reach agreement on expectations.

    - Lab and x-ray establish turnaround guarantees for ED (HCAB 1999).

34. Stop tampering. Analyze the process and redesign it instead of using a "Band-Aid."

35. Use differentiation.

36. Reduce the number of components.

37. Apply default mode (only one way).

38. Reduce controls on the system. (Rather than using eight inspection points, identify the first inspection point, redesign it to 99% effectiveness, and eliminate the seven other inspection points, improving quality, decreasing patient dissatisfaction while waiting for the eight inspections, and decreasing cost of inspection.)

39. Reduce classifications.

40. Synchronize. Time all steps in a process with reference to a clearly defined, agreed-upon synchronization point.

    - Make the synchronization point for surgery the incision time.

– Make the synchronization point for ambulatory care the moment when the physician walks into the examining room.

– Make the synchronization point for inpatient admission the moment the ED physician determines the patient needs to be admitted (not when the admitting physician communicates admitting orders).

41. Schedule into multiple processes.

    – Rather than a one-size-fits-all process, use multiple versions of the process, each tailored to the different needs of customers or users.

    – Use a separate process for ED patients with less serious conditions.

    – Use a separate process for ED patients with extremity injuries.

42. Minimize handoffs.

    – Have the same staff perform multiple functions. Train staff to perform tasks, answer questions versus having to ask for another staff or supervisor to intervene and write procedures to avoid delays from staff intervention lag time.

    – In ED, provide ED physician access to x-ray before radiologist reading complete versus waiting on radiologist (HCAB 1999).

    – Assign hospitalists to manage inpatient care, particularly to expedite ED admissions (HCAB 1999).

43. Consider people to be in the same system. Take steps to help people see themselves as part of the same system working toward a common aim.

    – Consider the surgeon's office and hospital to be parts of the same system.

    – See all processes leading to surgery as parts of the same system. (See also Synchronize, number 40.)

    – Incorporate ED and floor nurses as parts of the same system by organizing joint management teams.

    – Incorporate imaging, lab, and ED as parts of the same system by including them in ED improvement activities.

– Assign dedicated x-ray and phlebotomist staff in ED (HCAB 1999).

44. Use multiple processing units.

– Use several small centrifuges instead of one large centrifuge.

– Designate an alternate site for subspecialty patients.

– To optimize patient care throughput, provide an extended short-stay recovery unit for outpatient surgery and procedures requiring extended recovery times instead of using inpatient capacity (HCAB 2002).

45. Adjust to peak and trough demand. (Graph staffing by hour to demand by hour and increase staffing at peak, decrease staffing at troughs. Avoid 12-hour shifts unless demand curve operates in 12-hour increments [rare]).

46. Use pull systems. When work is being transferred through a process, instead of "pushing" it from one step to the next, have the later step "pull" it from the previous step.

– Pull patients from ED to inpatient unit. The Be-a-Bed-Ahead system addresses the delay in moving patients from one point of care to the next—for example, from the ED to the inpatient unit or to ICU. Delays occur between the time when ED staff notify receiving units that a patient requires a bed and the time the patient is actually transferred. The call from ED triggers a chain of events that eventually leads to the patient being transported to the unit. Under a Be-a-Bed-Ahead system, the inpatient units and ICU anticipate the demand (by measuring demand over time) and have a bed ready into which a patient can be moved ("pulled" versus "pushed") as soon as an ED patient needs a bed.

– Assign ED a set number of beds per hour, based on 80% statistically determined demand from ED.

– Pull asthma patients from ED to the primary care site. Asthma patients seen in the ED are often told to make an appointment at a primary care site for follow-up care. However, many patients simply do not make the appointments. In the redesign, the primary care clinic establishes a pull system by having slots available so that the staff in the ED can make the appointment for the patient before the patient leaves the ED.

– Pull patients from ED triage into an ED bed by giving the triage nurse, instead of the ED RN, access to and control of ED bed placement.

47. Give people access to information.

– Measure and post ED physician profiles (HCAB 1999).

48. Coach customers to use product/service.

49. Use a coordinator and expeditor.

– In ED, deploy dedicated communications nurse (HCAB 1999).

50. Optimize the level of inspection.

51. Reduce setup or startup time.

– Use preformatted charting (HCAB 1999).

52. Standardize.

– Use identical room setups for surgery.

53. Develop operational definitions.

– Define "ED visit" to end when a request for an inpatient bed is entered into the system instead of when the patient is transported to the patient care unit. Assign control from "request for bed" until inpatient bed to the inpatient unit manager. ED managers do not control when the patient bed is assigned; unit managers do.

54. Improve predictions.

– Predict periods of high ED demand.

– Use predictions of demand to set panel sizes and staffing.

– Predict demand for same-day appointments.

55. Use visual controls and reminders.

– Design the ED tracking system so that the patient's name flashes at 45 minutes into the stay to prompt the nurse to ensure that all diagnostic tests have been ordered by the ED physician.

56. Use constraints and forcing functions.

57. Use affordances.

58. Use redundancy, when appropriate.

59. Offer product/service anytime.

60. Offer product/service anyplace.

61. Convert internal steps to external. Convert tasks that are done as part of the process to tasks that are performed ahead of time or deferred until later.

    – Have standardized doses available ahead of time.

    – Move consultations from ED to inpatient setting.

    – Customize central supplies for particular physicians.

MATCH STAFFING AND CAPACITY TO DEMAND

62. Match inventory to predicted demand.

63. Invest more resources in improvement.

    – Convert case manager time from 75% inspection work (Cost of Quality) to 75% improvement work (that is, instead of inspecting, case managers are trained to design care processes so that inspection is not necessary).

64. Redefine the resource "cell" to optimize capacity.

    – Optimize surgery team utilization rather than OR suite utilization.

    – ED team versus assigning teams to specific ED rooms.

    – Patient care team versus assigning teams to specific inpatient room blocks.

65. Balance centralized and decentralized capacity.

    – Use centralized staff to meet fluctuations in demand at the local level.

    – Use centralized staff in high-demand periods.

66. Work down the backlog.

    – If the system has accumulated a backlog, add some capacity in the short term to reduce the backlog.

- Take on additional work in the short term.

- Use additional providers in the short term.

67. Cross-train centralized staff.

68. Focus on core processes and purpose.

69. Share risks.

70. Develop alliance/cooperative relationships.

71. Mass customize and standardize.

72. Adjust to peak and trough demand.

    - Match physicians' schedules with patient demand.

    - Adjust ED staff to periods of predictably high demand with innovatively varied start-end shifts versus traditional staffing paradigms (and decrease during predictably low demand).

73. Reduce demotivating aspects of pay system.

74. Conduct training.

75. Implement cross-training.

76. Emphasize natural and logical consequences.

SHAPE DEMAND

77. Optimize maintenance.

78. Promote self-care. Create or reveal the capacity of patients to treat themselves.

    - Provide nebulizer therapy at home.

    - Use diagnostic testing at home.

    - Teach in-home otoscope use.

79. Anticipate the demand. Meet a need before it arises.

    - Give breastfeeding instruction prior to discharge.

    - Have cardiac nurse visit patient at home preoperatively.

80. Relocate the demand.

    - Administer immunizations in school.

 – Have LPNs remove sutures.

 – Schedule lunch-hour checkups.

81. Automate. Meet a recurrent need with a standardized process.

 – Answer clinical questions via audiotape or Internet.

82. Extinquish demand for ineffective care.

 – Minimize treatment that has no evidence of efficacy. In its *Guide to Clinical Preventive Services* (1996), the U.S. Preventive Services Task Force reports on more than 200 commonly performed preventive practices and finds a lack of scientific evidence for many of them.

 – Allow longer intervals between camp physicals.

 – In ED, eliminate unnecessary tests through ordering guidelines (HCAB 1999).

 – In ED, profile ED physician use of ancillary services (HCAB 1999).

83. Combine services. Reframe the original demand for individualized service into a large cluster of services.

 – Group appointments for patients with hypertension.

84. Insert an information delay. Postpone immediate service for the specific purpose of obtaining information from the waiting period.

 – Wait for conditions to improve with time. For example, the parent of a toddler requests an appointment to have the febrile child examined. The nurse practitioner predicts that the child's upper respiratory infection should improve within two days and suggests that the parent bring the child in after two days if he is not improved.

 – Educate patients during waiting times.

Disclaimer: Neither ASQ, Chip Caldwell & Associates nor its representatives can recommend the efficacy, safety, or appropriateness of any change. The organization's leadership must assume full responsibility and accountability for using this research.

REFERENCES

Caldwell, Chip, and Charles Denham. 2001. *Medication Safety and Cost Recovery.* Chicago: Health Administration Press.

Clinical Initiatives Center. 2002. *Optimizing CCU Throughput.* Washington: Advisory Board Company.

Healthcare Advisory Board. 1999. *The Clockwork ED.* Washington: Advisory Board Company.

————. 2002. *Maximizing Hospital Capacity: Expediting Patient Throughput in an Era of Shortage.* Washington: Advisory Board Company.

Nolan, Thomas, et al. 1996. *Reducing Delays and Waiting Times.* Boston: Institute for Healthcare Improvement.

U.S. Preventive Services Task Force. 1996. *Guide to Clinical Preventive Services.* Baltimore: Williams & Williams.

Appendix D

PDCA Project Method Assessment Workpaper

Rank each discipline according to its effectiveness (5 represents "high performance" and 1 represents "low performance"). Record interventions to close obvious gaps.

PDCA step	Discipline	Score	Intervention (if any)
P	1. Strategically-aligned mission/charter.		
	2. Use of SMART-type form.		
	3. Process discovery tool effectiveness.		
	a. Look for flowchart, spreadsheet, or other method of listing sequential steps, rework loops, wait loops, dependencies, and other factors critical to process understanding. Unacceptable responses include "We brainstormed how the process works, but didn't write it down" or "We know how the process works."		
	b. Look for a baseline measure reflecting current performance that is linked to the mission/charter metric.		
	4. Process root cause analysis. Look for evidence that the manager collected data (as opposed to simply "gut feel" or pre-determined bias) to uncover the subprocesses and factors driving the most variation. Acceptable tools include cause and effect/fishbone, spreadsheet listing, Pareto chart, and so on. Tools that examine subprocess metrics and categories such as people, process, policy, plant/equipment, environment/legal are acceptable.		

Continued

183

Continued

PDCA step	Discipline	Score	Intervention (if any)
	5. Creative process intervention. Look for evidence that the team created an intervention criteria selection matrix first and, second, brainstormed a list of at least five potential interventions from which to pilot. An unacceptable response is, "We knew what we wanted to try so we didn't need to discuss other alternatives."		
D	6. Active experimentation. Look for evidence that the team considered the intervention as a pilot and structured a time-limited evaluation period. Use of metrics is a prerequisite to a high score; no metrics, other than anecdotal, results in a score of 1.		
C	7. Response to experiment and conclusions.		
A	8. Hold the gains processes. If the pilot is successful upon analysis of the data in step C, did the team transfer the intervention to operating units? Evidence would include a revised policy, introduction of training, and/or deployment of a department-based Quality Control Spreadsheet or Failure Modes and Effects Analysis (FMEA) spreadsheet.		
A	9. PDCA Improvement. Did the team review the PDCA process they just completed and suggest one or more innovations to improve the PDCA process throughout the organization?		
	10. Speed. Did the team complete the PDCA in a rapid time frame (less than 90 days)?		
Six Sigma	11. Is there an opportunity to introduce Six Sigma tools into the PDCA process (such as FMEA, regression analysis, Lean-Six Sigma Solution Sets, and so on)?		

Index

About the Authors

Chip Caldwell is the president of Chip Caldwell & Associates, and is formerly senior vice president of Premier Performance Services and Health Industry Executive of Juran Institute. He specializes in strategic deployment of clinical and systems quality improvement and cost reduction initiatives in medical centers, extended care facilities, integrated health systems, and health plans. Caldwell previously served as president of the HCA Atlanta health system, an eight hospital network with fifteen owned family practice centers and over 250 contracted physicians. He also served as president/CEO of HCA West Paces Medical Center in Atlanta from 1986 through 1993.

Jim Brexler is the CEO of Erlanger Health System of Chattanooga, Tennessee, a non-profit, academic teaching center affiliated with the University of Tennessee College of Medicine. Previously, Brexler was the vice chancellor of the Louisiana State University (LSU) Health Sciences Center and chief executive officer of the Health Care Services Division. Prior to the LSU posts, Brexler worked in executive capacities in healthcare institutions including Oakwood Healthcare System in Dearborn, Michigan; General Health System in Baton Rouge, Louisiana; and Greensboro Hospital in Greensboro, North Carolina.

Tom Gillem is a skilled communicator with expertise working along side senior leaders to shape both internal and external corporate messages, then disseminating the messages to appropriate audiences. His career includes daily newsgathering and reporting for more than two decades, political campaign work, media and public relations, executive consulting, teaching at the college level, developing quality/process improvement methodologies, and magazine editing and promotion projects. Most recently, he was Communications Manager at HealthLeaders Inc., Nashville, Tennessee, an integrated healthcare media and business information company.